Communication in Palliative Care

This practical, thought-provoking guide provides the unemotional, clear, and accurate advice necessary for communicating with patients in a palliative care setting – a pivotal aspect of being a palliative care expert that is so difficult to quantify and teach. It uses genuine anecdotes and case studies to bring theory to life and assist in everyday application.

The revised edition includes sections on the conversation about assisted dying and how it feels to be on the other side of clinical communication as a patient or carer.

Communication in Palliative Care is a wide-ranging, invaluable resource to palliative care professionals across all clinical settings.

Features:

- Offers the lessons learned over a lifetime of care in practice from diagnosis into bereavement
- Addresses the topics of daily concern to palliative care professionals and carers working in oncology or with non-malignant disease and with the elderly across all clinical settings
- Presents a succinct summary of points and lessons from each case study

Communication in Palliative Care

Clear Practical Advice, Based on a Series of Real Case Studies

Second Edition

Janet Dunphy

Retired Clinical Nurse Specialist & Teacher in Palliative Care
Retired Hospice Chief Executive
Current Independent Funeral Celebrant

Foreword by

Mary Kiely

Retired Consultant in Palliative Medicine, Huddersfield

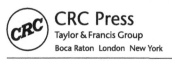

CRC Press
Taylor & Francis Group
Boca Raton London New York

CRC Press is an imprint of the
Taylor & Francis Group, an **informa** business

Designed cover image: Shutterstock

Second edition published 2025
by CRC Press
4 Park Square, Milton Park, Abingdon, Oxon, OX14 4RN

and by CRC Press
2385 NW Executive Center Drive, Suite 320, Boca Raton FL 33431

CRC Press is an imprint of Informa UK Limited

© 2025 Janet Dunphy

The right of Janet Dunphy to be identified as author of this work has been asserted in accordance with sections 77 and 78 of the Copyright, Designs and Patents Act 1988.

This book contains information obtained from authentic and highly regarded sources. While all reasonable efforts have been made to publish reliable data and information, neither the author[s] nor the publisher can accept any legal responsibility or liability for any errors or omissions that may be made. The publishers wish to make clear that any views or opinions expressed in this book by individual editors, authors or contributors are personal to them and do not necessarily reflect the views/opinions of the publishers. The information or guidance contained in this book is intended for use by medical, scientific or health-care professionals and is provided strictly as a supplement to the medical or other professional's own judgement, their knowledge of the patient's medical history, relevant manufacturer's instructions and the appropriate best practice guidelines. Because of the rapid advances in medical science, any information or advice on dosages, procedures or diagnoses should be independently verified. The reader is strongly urged to consult the relevant national drug formulary and the drug companies' and device or material manufacturers' printed instructions, and their websites, before administering or utilizing any of the drugs, devices or materials mentioned in this book. This book does not indicate whether a particular treatment is appropriate or suitable for a particular individual. Ultimately it is the sole responsibility of the medical professional to make his or her own professional judgements, so as to advise and treat patients appropriately. The authors and publishers have also attempted to trace the copyright holders of all material reproduced in this publication and apologize to copyright holders if permission to publish in this form has not been obtained. If any copyright material has not been acknowledged please write and let us know so we may rectify in any future reprint.

British Library Cataloguing-in-Publication Data
A catalogue record for this book is available from the British Library

ISBN: 978-1-032-54759-6 (hbk)
ISBN: 978-1-032-54757-2 (pbk)
ISBN: 978-1-003-42737-7 (ebk)

DOI: 10.1201/9781003427377

Typeset in Palatino
by SPi Technologies India Pvt Ltd (Straive)

To Dr Louise Jordan, with admiration, respect, and love; my friend, dedicated GP for Baslow, and pioneer for end-of-life services across North Derbyshire. The results of your passion are still felt and will always be remembered by those of us who were lucky enough to share your orbit. Your direct language and solution-orientated approach crashed down barriers and spread comfort. I will hear your laughter in my mind forever.

To Dawn, you taught me more than you will ever acknowledge. You deserve credit that you will never ask for. From your diagnosis, horrendous treatments, and palliative phase, you have lived with a level of positivity and selflessness, which is, I assure you, quite rare. You who have made me a better person, as a professional, you elevated my successes, you supported me to be the best version of myself. I will carry your love and philosophy with me always.

Contents

Foreword to the First Edition

It's 13 years since the first edition of this book was published, but I believe it remains as relevant now as then. Although I am now retired from clinical practice, my very recent experience in the NHS demonstrated to me that, sadly, many clinicians still don't communicate well with their patients. At a time when medical treatments are becoming more varied and more complex than ever, it behoves not only doctors but also the nurses and allied health professionals working alongside them to use language which is understood by their patients when negotiating treatment options as well as foster an ethos of shared decision-making in an era of realistic medicine.

There has also been a change in society's attitudes over this time, and many people both anticipate and expect that more and more treatments will be available and on offer right up to and including the very end of life, even when those treatments offer little, if any, benefit to the sickest patients. Courage and honesty remain, therefore, ever more important qualities for clinicians, and when combined with kindness and compassion can produce conversations and ultimately decisions which truly honour a patient's wish for a good death.

Mary Kiely
Retired Consultant in Palliative Medicine, Huddersfield

Foreword to the Second Edition

They say that the genius of Mozart and Bill Gates isn't actually in their genes, but in the 10,000 hours plus that they each spent honing their craft. It really is true that practice makes perfect, or at least very good. They also say that you can't actually teach someone good communication skills – that either you've got it or you haven't.

Janet Dunphy has spent well over 10,000 hours doing what she does, communicating sensitive and life-transforming information to patients and their families, and she is very, very good at what she does.

Not only is Janet a highly experienced clinical nurse specialist and an exceptional communicator, but she also has the added skill of being able to break down the constituent parts of what makes a good patient–professional interaction and transform them into meaningful prose that brings alive the conversations with patients who are approaching the end of life.

A large part of the working week of a specialist palliative care professional is taken up with the education of others, either informally through clinical interaction or by way of formal or didactic teaching. Over almost 12 years, I have worked alongside Janet in both hospital and community palliative care teams. In clinical interactions and in our joint participation in formal teaching sessions, I have seen first-hand her consummate skills in assessing a clinician, reading an audience, and making the theory of education chime with the reality of the day-to-day practice of looking after patients at the end of life.

Janet appreciates that one of the most important attributes of a good teacher is familiarity with one's specialist area and the ability to demonstrate a passion and conviction for it. Often, 'experts' who have become removed from clinical practice, by the necessity of academic or management pressures, lose some of this passion or are so far removed from the day-to-day grindstone that their advice and guidance lack validity. As a still-active clinical nurse specialist, Janet can speak and write with the conviction of her expertise.

Sometimes the only way to learn how to do something is to see someone else do it several times and then keep doing it yourself until competent. Sadly, and particularly within the healthcare professions, this 'learning on the job' is increasingly seen as less valuable or relevant than formal lectures, personal reading, reflective analysis, and other more formal activities. But in busy clinical settings, it can be difficult, if not impossible, to get the chance to observe enough significant conversations between experienced clinicians and their patients to improve one's own skills and learn 'from the experts'. This is particularly the case when patients are very ill, and the discussions as crucial as those relating to end-of-life care.

There are lots of books about communication skills, but many are often no more than simple instruction manuals. Many books may indeed tell you what you need to do, but having read them, you will be no wiser as to why that is what you need to do. Janet's skill in this book lies in her ability to combine theory with narrative, and natural science with humanity, to create a text that resonates deeply. It is her ability to put into writing those attributes ideally gleaned from observing an expert clinician which makes this book special.

It is often said that experts make the difficult, or even the impossible, look effortless when, in reality, there is a lot of hard graft out of sight, the frantic undercarriage of the serenely calm swan. It is these efforts that Janet is able to articulate for the reader, bringing to light the message that intellectual knowledge is nothing if not accompanied by sensitive delivery and humanity.

Mary Kiely
Retired Consultant in Palliative Medicine, Huddersfield

About the Author

Janet Dunphy qualified as a nurse in 1980. She has spent over 30 years working, studying, and teaching as a clinical nurse specialist in palliative care. Her clinical experience spans both the NHS and voluntary sector and includes hospital and community roles.

Latterly, Janet was a hospice chief executive, dealing with austerity measures, the pandemic, and a merger. Her greatest success in this role was developing and implementing hospice-at-home services and volunteer community support services.

Currently, she enjoys her role as an independent funeral celebrant.

Janet is passionate about the future of palliative care services and education; her academic background is in communication and ethics. She cares deeply about how people die and improving the services to support the patient, their loved ones, and the bereaved. Janet continues to study and, most of all, listen to and learn from the stories of ordinary people.

Acknowledgements

I am grateful to the following people:

To Dr Mary Kiely, Consultant in Palliative Medicine, now retired – my esteemed colleague, friend, and debating opponent. Thank you for sharing your wonderful mind with me, for the teaching, for learning, and for thinking that I should write books. Your time is so precious, and yet you invest in me. You will always be my guru, the oracle. Thank you so much for your wisdom, pedantry, and patience. May we teach and walk through graveyards together until we drop; chances are that we will, and I love and appreciate it all.

To Marian – whose intelligence, thoughtfulness, and loyalty sustained me over many years. This book would not have happened without your time and integrity. You are and always will be a very special person in my life and one of my greatest treasures. I have so much pleasure knowing that you know this.

To Joan and Christine – you believed in me, and my ability to write, wholeheartedly. When I wavered, your belief did not. It is because of your knowledge of writing and publishing that I felt my confidence grow as I worked and because of you that I felt this book was even possible. Thank you sincerely.

To all the patients and their loved ones, to all the bereaved families who shared their stories – you touched my life, altered my shape, and taught me everything. I have been humbled and sustained by your presence in my world. Metaphorically I nod towards you here, with warmth and the deepest of respect and thanks, for all that you were and all that you are.

1

Introduction: A Note from the Author

As a retired nurse, educator, and chief executive (I am 64 years old, by the way), I have spent a lot of time talking, teaching, and sharing my experience and like so many nurses, I can tell a good story, which has proved useful as my current role is an independent funeral celebrant. I now have the privilege of being able to listen to and tell the life stories of others. My learning and passion for how we communicate as professionals and the effect we have on people's lives and deaths have only increased over time.

The Educational Value of Telling the Story

The preceding paragraph is revealing: my age, professions, and one of my passions – education. This introduction is just for that reason: to allow you as the reader to get to know me a bit and understand why I wrote this book. It is my chance to talk to you about my experience, style, and why I think those stories are more important than ever. Historically, under the pressures of academic work and essay writing, we lost the knack of sharing them. We all have those stories inside us and sharing them is a valuable educational tool. Across healthcare, the quality and safety frameworks have embedded the value of collating and sharing the lessons of patient experience in their frameworks. The value of audits and clinical reviews is now part of the architecture in health and social care.

Everything Changes

We have all seen the pressures change in healthcare. Change is a certainty. Everything changes and healthcare definitely has, massively. It has changed to meet the demands of biological and sociological developments. The advances in information technology and the systems we use have radically changed how we send and receive information.

The COVID-19 pandemic wrought changes across the world, most keenly felt in health and social care. As professionals we saw improvements in systems and practice delivered at speed, bureaucracy moved quickly to the benefit of all. Such technological advances are indeed positive but must be balanced, in my opinion, with remembering that we are in 'the people business'. Kindness and clarity have never been more important. My assertion is that, in terms of communication, our priority and purpose has not changed. The more complex healthcare becomes, the more important it is to keep to the simple rules.

DOI: 10.1201/9781003427377-1

We are each a product of our experiences, and 43 years of motherhood and working alongside the dying and bereaved have inevitably shaped the way I think. I have been fortunate; I knew, as a child, that I wanted to be a nurse and, as a student nurse, that I wanted to work with dying patients. Those were my thoughts back then. Palliative care as a specialty had not been born, but I had a strong sense of where I belonged, and I have kept it simple.

Case Studies and Conversations

My aim is to do the same with my writing, to explore key contemporary issues, to describe the necessary skills, and to use thought-provoking case studies from genuine experiences. For the sake of integrity, and with respect to the reader, the context stays within my experience as a nurse in the UK and acknowledges that not all issues are covered in depth. I know how hard all healthcare professionals work and how many are involved on a daily basis in providing good palliative care. It is my intention that you all feel that my work here relates to and is useful to you, whatever your job and wherever you do it. There are better paid and less stressful jobs, but making the difference to palliative care patients has to be one of the most rewarding. It would be difficult to sustain if it wasn't: it would cost too much emotionally. Effective communication is just one aspect of this worthwhile job. Modern systems now ensure that service user feedback is integral to evaluation and shaping services for the future. We encourage the service user's voice and promote personalisation and personal choices; this book aims to support those initiatives.

Twenty-five Years' Experience

I first worked in a UK hospice in the 1980s and started the studies that all nurses engage in and endure. I realised how much I did not know and studied harder before progressing to be a Macmillan specialist nurse in palliative care, working from a hospital oncology unit and covering community. By then, I had also learnt that I loved teaching and that, in healthcare, we study forever, in some form or other. Colleagues would tell you that I am a natural teacher, but I have never forgotten the basics, the reason why we do our job and why we study and share our experience: the patient and their carers. Of course, I know the academic terms and clichés, but I know also that the case studies and genuine clinical anecdotes will be as helpful to the reader.

As my career moved on, I changed my place and clinical area of work, but for most of my career I stayed with the patients. I was a clinical nurse specialist in palliative care for 25 years and have worked in and out of hospices, in community with the general practitioners (GPs) and community nurses, in hospitals on the wards with the doctors, nurses, and other staff and in nursing/care homes.

Since the first edition in 2011 life has changed for me too, as you would expect. I moved from clinical practice into senior management, chief executive of a hospice, a hospice which merged successfully with another community end-of-life care provider during the battles of the COVID-19 pandemic – a pandemic which shook the foundations of the world and every provider of health and social care. Using the measurable elements of quality, volume and finance I was successful in the role. And yet, something was missing for me: my personal reward system – patient/family contact – it's just who I am.

During that part of my career, I also moved my elderly parents in with me to provide them with love and care in their final years. They lived with me for 4.5 years and died at home with me at the ages of 96 and 94. Together, we coped with the effects of ageing and the deterioration of every physiological process, which sadly included dementia. Some assumed that I had all the competencies to deal with that, but as you may know yourselves, nothing quite prepares you for how hard it is; it was yet another steep learning curve for me.

After 7.5 years in the post, I retired and returned with glee to the community to work with a diverse range of families to provide personalised funeral services. It felt like a natural progression, to be involved in the final part of life's journey with dedicated professionals in a new sector. It is after all the final phase of palliative/end-of-life care practice. Every interaction from diagnosis leads to this point, where experiences, grievances, sadness, and joy meet to enable the memorialisation of someone to be both meaningful and therapeutic. It is a place and time where stories are told, and you know how much I love stories and appreciate their value in education.

There are only 2 days in our lives that are less than 24 hours long; the day we are born and the day we die. The former is celebrated annually, and the latter is dealt with quickly and usually with civic formality and, sadly, with little planning or discussion. The final chapter in this edition hopes to redress the balance. After a long career in palliative, end-of-life, and bereavement care, I know the arenas we work in, and I know how to write about it.

We Are Patients and Carers Too

Being a professional and patient or a carer can be tricky to navigate. As a professional, it can be tricky to communicate with a patient or carer who is also a professional. In this grey area can lie unreasonable expectations of other carers, unfair responsibilities, frustrations and tears. It can add another layer of stress to an already anxious time. It's a challenge that doesn't seem to be mentioned or taught, so I have included a chapter on this. The memory of an unsatisfactory experience can last a lifetime; like most difficult events, it isn't something we consider before it happens to us.

We Mustn't Lose the Knack of Laughing

I also believe that compassion is an easy bedfellow with humour – they can be synergistic. Sometimes I worry that as professionals, we have become bogged down and have lost the knack of laughing and sharing our stories. We are regularly taught the science of what we do, the models and the theories, and that is crucial. What we are rarely taught and do not acknowledge even to ourselves is the 'art' in what we do. Some things cannot be taught; some skills are part of our personality. Those skills, however, can be identified and developed, and it is often those skills that take us from being the learner to the confident practitioner.

I hope as you read that you can identify with the art I describe and that you stop to pat yourself on the back as an ordinary person with special attributes who has chosen to journey alongside those who suffer.

The format of this book describes the journey for the patient and their carers, and as they often share the same experience, I have not separated their feelings. The content will apply to all professionals in healthcare, and I use the umbrella term *professional* to respect all disciplines. For simplicity and gender continuity, I will use the pronoun *she* for the professional and *he* for the patient. The word *client* is only used when funerals (which, of course, are paid for) and bereavement support are being discussed.

Many Different Settings

As professionals, we see our patients go through the phases of illness and experience a variety of clinical settings, getting used to many medical terms along the way. The term *clinical setting* applies to the place of care for the patient. This changes from home and the care of the GP and community nurse to hospital, perhaps as an outpatient or as an inpatient under the care of clinical teams of doctors and nurses. Care homes and hospices may also be a vital part of the patient's journey. It is for this reason that I talk of all settings to acknowledge and support all professionals working in all places of care. Our hospices are undoubtedly centres of excellence, but a hospice is not a building; it is a philosophy, which has been successfully transferred to other settings such as the patients' homes and on hospital wards where marvellous high-standard care is often provided. As a specialist nurse, I learnt early on that we are not special, we just specialise, and I have been lucky enough to work alongside so many inspirational professionals from pathologists to funeral directors.

Whilst the bulk of my clinical experience has been with cancer patients, the patient suffering from non-malignant disease endures identical problems and often has fewer resources allocated to them. My messages here are therefore not cancer-specific as excellent communication is needed whatever the clinical diagnosis. As we treat and manage disease more effectively, we must ensure that good communication is not prescribed in subtherapeutic doses, because in palliative care, it may be the only prescription available.

As people live longer, the ageing population increases its demands on services. The figures for dementia sufferers rise as people's life expectancy increases. I have evolved to accept the science of ageing and dying that, as biological machines, we collect chronic diseases as we age and then we die. We do not 'pass away', 'get lost', or 'go to sleep'; we die, and dying matters. We do it only once. I have not become blasé or hard; I am just as soft as I was and proud of it too. However, I have got stronger and accepted that I cannot fix everything, and ensured that my patients and their families know this, but that I can make an unforgettable difference at the worst of times. With this knowledge, let us be brave and use grown-up words like *death* and *dying*.

Whilst the public expects more from us, we know that we can only treat and manage most diseases. Cure applies only to some infections and some cancers. Everything else we can only manage whether it is diabetes, heart disease, or liver disease. It is the management of dealing with people and disease that requires both art and science.

Three Score Years and Ten

When I recall my student days, I remember the phrase 'three score years and ten'. Patients and families meant they had enjoyed what was then termed 'a good innings'. Conversely, today we are more used to hearing sentences start with the phrases, 'You would think in this day and age ...' or 'With all the technology today ...'. These statements are just as frequently applied to patients older than their 'three score years and ten'. Middle-aged people are now often saying, 'Why my dad?' not 'Well, he has had his three score years and ten'. The population is living longer and expecting more. A baby born today in most places in the developed world will have an average life expectancy of 81.5 years in comparison to 1960 when it was 66.8 for men and 73.2 for women.

Today's Patient

Information is more accessible and transferrable electronically than ever. Most of our patients use the internet, read, or search for information in some way. The public is hungry for answers and more confident about asking questions of the professionals caring for them.

One percent of the population will die each year; in the UK, this means 600,000. The average UK GP has approximately 25 dying people on their practice list at any one time. Contemporary politics has supported us since the UK Department of Health's publication of the *End of Life Care Strategy* in 2008.[1]

Many white papers have been published since then, and all demonstrate the value of death awareness, advance care planning, early and sensitive discussions and improved services. We must therefore be honest and clear in our dialogue. The increasing number of questions and thirst for knowledge demand this, and if we cannot have open discussions using the appropriate words, how can we change from being a death-denying society to a society that cares for and talks to each other as we die? The 21st-century patient is not the compliant soul of yesteryear. Euphemisms and platitudes belong in history. The modern patient negotiates their information needs and demands much more from the professionals caring for them.

As a society, we have seen an increased profile for assisted dying. It is a topic that will be mentioned sometimes by those in our care and can be uncomfortable to discuss. I have therefore included a chapter on this to support those tricky discussions. Importantly, I want to support all professionals who have those discussions to ensure that they leave these discussions feeling confident that the issue was dealt with kindly, professionally, and clearly.

Death has been taken from the closet and slapped on the table. Most people do actually want to talk about it. They want to discuss everything: symptoms, diagnosis, treatment, prognosis, feelings, and coping strategies. All problems are lessened or solved by communication, from minor disagreements to international war. Given the expectations of our society, we need to be skilled and confident to meet them. I think that it is the least we can do.

All clinical areas have escalating stress factors, now more than ever. Every professional, in my opinion, deserves to feel proud of their professional and personal investment into every working day. This book aims to help in achieving that.

Reference

1. Department of Health. *End of Life Care Strategy: Promoting high quality care for all adults at the end of life*. Cm 9840. London: Department of Health; 2008.

2

Relationships

Who is the most important person in your life?

Everyone would answer the preceding question differently, and when faced with a new patient, professionals have little or no idea of the patient's or carer's values and experiences, and everyone is a product of their experiences. It would be extremely valuable to society if the subject of relationships were taught in the school curriculum. Everyone has them, and all too often, people bring significant gaps in information and skills to their later relationships. Relationships are formative – pivotal issues that shape and define us. Quite simply, they make professionals who they are and, more importantly, they make their patients and their carers who they are.

Fifty-four per cent of carers have left their jobs to care,[1] and 2.6 million people have reduced work or given up work to care for elderly or seriously unwell family members because of caring responsibilities.[2] The care they provide is unpaid. The standard current carer's allowance in the UK is £76.75 per week. The mental and emotional cost is immeasurable. Additionally, 60% of carers report a long-term health condition or disability compared to 50% of non-carers.[3]

We know that many people seen in healthcare services are also carers and that loved ones often take the strain off the NHS services, and it's the strain that it is so important to acknowledge and plan for. NHS services are overloaded; social care struggles to meet demand, so it's important to be clear and realistic about what support is available and discuss that services can only fill the gaps left by family and friends who are caring for the patient at home. Outside of hospital and residential care, there is no such thing as 24-hour care available from the NHS and social care. Family and social constructs are often complex, professionals can't assume who the main carer may be. It helps to ask openly and agree to direct advice and information to that person. This is especially helpful in big families. The financial burden of caring and loss of income is huge for many people. A referral to services that support carers and advice regarding benefits is crucial and should be made early in the clinical relationship when appropriate.

The impact of how relationships past and present affect people cannot be overestimated. The range of normal reactions is wide. People display a huge variety of personal responses. Family dynamics often play an important part in our relationships and will underpin many of our reactions. A close happy family will often react with strong emotions, and their sense of loss will be immense.

Conversely, where a family member has been estranged or had a difficult relationship with another family member, there will also be a strong reaction.

The only safe assumption is that it is not safe to assume anything. With all this in mind, professionals have to evaluate their patients and form a therapeutic relationship, usually at the worst of times for the patient and their carers. They have to communicate effectively with all other professionals involved and be aware of their own 'personal triggers' – the

DOI: 10.1201/9781003427377-2

situations that they may face that have a personal meaning to them and therefore may elicit a personal and emotional response.

Remember the question at the start of this chapter. Professionals are often faced with emotive situations and family dynamics very close to their own experience and these form the 'personal triggers'. Sometimes they are easily identified and planned for, and at other times, such triggers appear unexpectedly; they can sneak under the professional's radar and become an added difficulty and complexity in the patient–professional relationship. In healthcare, professionals move from task to task, tasks that involve people, where one person's life touches another's.

CLAIRE'S STORY

I am 48 years old and an experienced clinical nurse specialist working in a busy hospital. I love my job, and I am still confident after doing it for 20 years. So, the referral for an elderly man in the dying phase of his illness was not a particular challenge to me. I knew the care of the elderly ward and its staff well. It did not seem a clinically complex case, and on paper, Eddie seemed to be dying peacefully from his metastatic prostate cancer. I had been asked just to pop in and check that all his care was okay.

I arrived on the ward, enjoyed my usual friendly chat with the staff and walked into Eddie's side room. Eddie was unconscious, peaceful, and obviously well cared for, but that wasn't the first visual impact. It was the small, elegant, meek-mannered lady sat at the back of his room; she sat (both in her body language and chosen position in the room) as although she didn't want to be in the way. She was perfectly groomed, with earrings, clothes, shoes, scarf, and handbag all matching. Her expression was gentle, unassuming, and accepting of the pain of loss that lay before her.

I sat with her to hear her story of how much she loved Eddie and had since they were 20 years old. They had done everything together, no separate interests, an old-fashioned marriage of 58 years that had worked. They had raised a family together. Eddie had worked as an engineer and managed all the technical aspects of running a house; the television controller was a mystery to Dora, his wife, who had cooked, cleaned, and organised all the housekeeping and bills.

They were a real partnership and loyal friends. He was the love of her life, and she was watching him die without anger or frustration. She was philosophical: 'It happens to us all you know, love', she whispered as though she was preparing me, the younger woman who hadn't been on this earth as long and had much to learn about loving and letting go.

She had no concerns or questions; she accepted the scene before her with grace and humility. She was full of praise for the staff and thanked me for my visit: 'You have a lovely kind face, love', she told me, and she tapped my hand, as if to say, 'It's okay now, love; all is well here'.

I left the room and didn't stop to talk to the staff as I normally do because I was crying, quietly, huge tears pouring down my face as I walked through the busy ward. To me, that could have been my mum and dad. I could imagine them being that way. My mum is so like that lady, and I know she too would be the elegant, accepting, meek-mannered lady who sat quietly as her soulmate left her, and it had hit me hard, just for a while, and I hadn't seen it coming.

> It was a good experience, and I learnt from it. I rang to feed back to the staff and my reaction was one that they respected and understood because it can happen to all of us. We reflect and then we grow as professionals. I am glad that I met Eddie and Dora and hope that amidst the saddest moment of her life, Dora knew that she had been in the presence of someone who cared. It was all that was needed that day.

There is much to learn and acknowledge by considering Claire's story. It puts the meat on the bones of the phrase 'personal triggers'. The lessons learnt from the story can be understood and transferred to other situations common to professionals. Everyone has a family, people they care for, a history, a valuable story unique to them yet often compatible with others. Sometimes, professionals can see the triggers at the time of written or verbal referral, and they have time to adjust their emotions before meeting the patient, and sometimes they are adjusting whilst in the situation, whilst being the kind professional, and it's hard. It is important to acknowledge that – it is hard. If professionals seek to be a decent human being, first and foremost, and a decent professional, second, they do not go far wrong. Staying human and being in the experience with the patient and his carers is fundamental to the success of all interactions. That way, those in need feel safe, understood, and cared for.

It is important to note that the term *caring* is not being used in a self-sacrificing, virtuous way. Caregiving is a complex concept, which includes assessment, intricate thought processes, instinct, experience, skill, and knowledge. It is not merely the altruistic act of a 'nice person'. Professionals are poor at defining what it is to be caring; this is something that all professionals need to acknowledge to themselves to increase self-worth and define more accurately to their managers and the public to increase understanding of their roles.

The interaction with Dora involved an assessment of Dora's (and, it can be assumed, Eddie's) value system. By listening and being present in the moment, Claire made a valuable connection with Dora, who quickly shared personal and helpful information with her. Claire was therefore able to understand the relationship that Dora had with the patient and provide meaningful support whilst assessing the patient's symptoms and care plan. She established a relationship of trust in an emotional environment. Dora was not aware of her sadness, but she was aware and grateful for her kindness – that's the skill, right there, in that short visit to the ward; that's the art and science of caring.

Dora trusted Claire enough to share precious memories and insights, foundational experiences, and information that led Claire's responses. She was not leading with emotions; she was leading with her intellect whilst being a caring human being. If caring was all that was needed for a professional–patient and carer relationship, anyone could do it and they can't; it takes so much more than just being caring. This is discussed in more depth in the next chapter. It is also obvious from Claire's story how respectful she was to the staff and how supportive they were of her. Those relationships are not built overnight. They take enormous skill and lots of time to develop to be an effective clinical relationship. All healthcare environments have complex hierarchies, often fraught with difficulties. The medical model is still alive and well. Decisions and treatment plans are, often appropriately, made solely by the doctor. Yet all professionals are involved in the assessment and interventions needed to support patients and their carers. The relationships and dynamics can be complicated, difficult, and time-consuming to understand. Successful interactions are a challenge. All professionals have their own language, and they all feel that theirs is the most important language. Yet communicating with others is vital if clinical care is to be effective. It is true that respect is earned, it is not a given, and it takes being a professional.

TIP: The most important resource a professional brings to the situation is herself.

References

1. *Carers Trust Social Care Survey, Carers Trust*, 2020.
2. *Juggling work and unpaid care, Carers UK*, 2019.
3. *Carers UK analysis of GP Patient Survey, Carers UK*, 2021.

3

Being a Professional

What is the difference between a lay carer and a professional?

The professional has a plan. They have been there before. They understand the continuum of disease affecting the patient. Whilst it isn't always possible to know where on the continuum each patient will be, a professional understands the prognostic indicators that a layperson doesn't see. They notice subtle messages, analyse the whole situation, utilise their knowledge, and make clinical plans.

It is these plans that make patients feel safe. A patient will meet many professionals of all disciplines throughout their journey. At times, they will be scared, very scared, desperate for information and, more importantly, for solutions. Palliative care is never about informing a patient that nothing more can be done; it's about what can be done. It is extremely difficult for vulnerable patients and their carers to receive often devastating clinical information and form a new relationship with a stranger. So, in these circumstances, how must a professional behave? Some of the behaviours are simple, possibly obvious; however, they are so crucial they are worth listing and considering. It is often the smallest things that are the most valuable when someone is vulnerable.

Confidence

Patients need to see and feel this from the beginning. It makes them feel safe at a time when the ground beneath them is shaking. Patients and their carers are in a position of need, hence the vulnerability, and when they meet professionals who act like they know what they are doing and have an air of confidence, they start to relax, listen, and take in vital information and form questions in their troubled minds. No one would want to ask a question of someone who didn't seem to know what they are doing. Whether buying a new computer, having a car fixed or getting a new mortgage, everyone will try to pick out the person who seems to be confident in their role. It makes a massive difference at the time when patients need it most. The aim is for the patient to be confident in the care they need and confident in the care providers. There are key professional characteristics that can create confidence.

Courtesy

This clearly demonstrates respect and kindness. It's so easy – a basic principle that ensures confidence in care. Courtesy is the first step in forming the clinical friendship that the patient will rely on throughout their journey. Courtesy isn't necessarily a formal thing;

DOI: 10.1201/9781003427377-3

good manners and respectful dialogue can easily be achieved using an informal style. The key here is timely and accurate assessment and negotiation, concepts which recur throughout this book. It is important to acknowledge that all public-sector workers have the skills and ability to make these assessments quickly, without realising that they are doing it. It's an innate skill that never sleeps. It is also inevitably used in family and social situations. No one can unknow what they know. Being professional isn't what you do: it's what you are.

PAULA'S STORY

My partner Ian's mum was a patient in the intensive care unit (ICU), having had a cardiac arrest during routine minor surgery. Ian is part of a big family, but they hadn't been in close contact over the years. The whole episode threw the family together in an understandable crisis. I hadn't met most of them and had to try to understand and support them at the worst of times for them. It's so hard to be the peripheral family member and a nurse. I chose to be quiet and respectful and support only if asked to do so. It was hard as they didn't see what I saw, and they didn't hear what I heard. I could see that they didn't understand what to me was obvious.

Ian's mum wouldn't recover; the machines and infusions were keeping her failing organs functioning, yet the family were hopeful and not ready to give up. I could see that they couldn't make sense of how a fit lady could now be so poorly in an ICU unit.

On Saturday (when Ian's mum had been in the ICU for 2 days), the whole family were there, going in to visit Ian's mum in twos. I sat waiting to go in with Ian and listened to each family member as they came back into the waiting room to tell of how well she looked today, that her colour had improved and her breathing was easier. I was both surprised and pleased to hear their accounts. Ian certainly was. Yet, when our turn came, I saw a completely different situation; I saw a dying lady, a dead lady essentially. I tried to answer my own questions: what was I seeing that the others didn't see? Her colour was awful; there was no elasticity in her skin; her breathing was centred in her upper abdomen, shallow and ineffective; her extremities were cold; and her nose was pinched. She was dying, soon.

I rejoined the family members and struggled to listen to their optimism. It wasn't my place to break bad news, and anyway, what if I was wrong? They didn't want an update from the ICU team. I felt as though I had the burden of a truth that they deserved to know more than me and that I had no right to be the one who told it to them. It was horrible, no one asked me questions, why would they? They were buoyant, chatting cheerfully and even planning to celebrate how well she looked. The burden of the obvious burned away inside me, and I struggled to find a way to do the right thing, what as a nurse I felt the right thing was. I decided a gentle warning shot would help, to say something that may prepare them and may make them think. It took courage to do it; this wasn't my mum in the bed, no one was asking for my opinion, yet I knew something that they didn't, just by seeing Ian's mum. I couldn't believe they saw something so completely different to me. I told them that Ian and I wouldn't be going out for a drink that evening in case we were called back. I wasn't in a position to be any more forceful than that. Of course, afterwards, I prepared

Ian for the worst, and we waited for the call I knew would come. Ian's mum died at 1 a.m., her family were shocked, and it was a dreadful time.

Bless Ian, the day after he filled the house with flowers for me and said he had watched me in awe with his family just always knowing what to say. It didn't feel like that to me. I just remember seeing something totally different than everyone else and that knowledge was a burden.

The knowledge that Paula felt as a burden in her personal life had taken years of experience to acquire, and when it's there, it never leaves. A professional can never be less than they are. Those skills of fast assessment and clinical knowledge enable a professional to establish a relationship quicker than a non-professional could. It is the accumulation of knowledge that enables a professional to notice what they see and give off that vital air of confidence that is so difficult to define and impossible to teach. Benner explains this well in her work regarding the move from novice to expert and states that '[t]he expert operates from a deep understanding of the total situation'.[1] It is this confidence and knowledge that help to promote trust. The patient–professional relationship has to be one of trust and establishing trust from the outset is a real challenge. It relies on some vital concepts such as truth telling, a pivotal issue and key confidence creator, which is discussed in more detail later.

A good professional is a kind professional, and a kind professional doesn't sympathise: they empathise. The difference between the two can be illustrated by the following analogy: if someone is stuck in a deep hole, a sympathetic person will get in the hole with them and feel what they feel; an empathetic person will see them in the hole, understand their feelings, and go for a ladder. All the skills and characteristics mentioned entail the professional sharing themselves, being human, negotiating with and connecting to a person in need, and using both informal and formal styles that display compassion and friendliness in equal measure. Yet patients are not the professional's friends; they have their own friends, so this is a relationship of professional responsibility. It is the responsibility that also divides the professional carer from the lay carer. Codes of conduct have to be adhered to. A professional is accountable for their practice and communication is a huge part of their practice.

The patient–professional relationship is transient; it is there when needed and should end when not needed. It is a contract of care, a privilege to be part of the patient's and their family's precious memories. To be involved at such treasured times is a real reward, one that professionals appreciate and learn from on a daily basis. Professionals walk alongside the living, not the dying. At the end of each working day, it takes skill and lots of experience to leave the thoughts attached to the patient and go home to another world, to be the mother, wife, or friend in a world devoid of the maelstrom of ever-increasing complexities in clinical practice. It takes adjustment, learning, and knowing how to let go to be ready for the next patient and their family, who will need the professional to act as though they are the only patients on their caseload to make the new patient feel unique, special, and safe.

Everyone in health and social care works within overloaded systems, and it's important to acknowledge that here. They work to targets, more and more of them, because new rules, guidance, and standards appear all the time. Many of the stresses faced are due to a lack of resources, and the stress caused gets passed to every attending clinician. It's vital to have coping strategies for professionals to remind yourself that they are only one part of the chain, and if their job is done well, that's all that they can do. Every professional finds their own way of 'leaving work behind' and that skill has become even more crucial when faced with an often frustrated public who have had to wait for an ambulance or an appointment, so many professional contacts have to start with listening to a story of stress caused by waiting (and even parking issues!). The consultation often now includes acknowledging what is being said, apologising for the impact and doing their own job well. Professionals are not responsible for every part of the system that the patient and the carer have been in contact with; they can only listen, acknowledge, and move on to do their own job kindly and politely; document everything clearly; and go off shift knowing that they could not have done more. Without such mantras, professionals would work in fear of complaints, investigations, and disciplinaries. In an overloaded and stressed workforce, this is too much to expect; to work with a fear of making a mistake can and often does become unbearable.

Self-care has never been needed more, having personal protection boundaries is absolutely necessary to be able to carry on working in a much-needed profession and survive.

Such adjustment takes years of experience to learn. Many mistakes are inevitably made along the way. It can be stressful, and stress can hurt. As the professional feels the pain, she will adjust, internalise what has happened and grow to be stronger and more empathetic than she was before. Professionals who block this process to avoid the hurt don't grow. They become stuck at the same level of understanding about the situation and themselves and stay as a novice, protecting themselves but helping far less than the professional who has been through the pain and adjustment, who has grown to understand themselves well, and who is always ready with compassion and confidence for the next patient, who will always come. The accomplished professional will take all past experiences and learning to the new patient and approach the first meeting with that vital confidence.

TIP: No one can unknow what they know.

Reference

1. Benner, P. *From Novice to Expert: Excellence and power in clinical nursing practice.* Menlo Park: Addison-Wesley; 1984. pp. 13–34.

4

Assessment Skills

People are taught to avert their eyes from abnormality; as professionals, we live in a world of abnormalities, and it's fascinating.

By definition, palliative care patients have been diagnosed with a life-threatening condition. Few people would want to be in that position. It is therefore worth trying to imagine what palliative care patients hope to experience as they sit waiting to meet the professional for the first time.

Dame Cicely Saunders's words set the scene well: 'You matter because you are you, and you matter to the end of your life. We will do all we can, not only to help you die peacefully, but also, to live until you die'.[1] Those inspirational words were supported formally by the World Health Organization when the definition of palliative care was first published in 1996:

'Palliative care is the active total care of patients whose disease is not responsive to curative treatment. Control of pain, of other symptoms and of psychological, social and spiritual problems is paramount. The goal of palliative care is [the] achievement of the best possible quality of life for patients and their families'.[2]

Amidst the many and various national and professional assessment models, palliative care assessments take their quality standards from those statements. The aim has to be total assessment, a consideration of all aspects of the patient, not merely the physical.

HARRY'S STORY

'A shadow' on my lung; could be anything, I thought. I'd been coughing all winter, but so have loads of other people. The GP sending me to the chest clinic, seemed a bit over the top to me, could have just given me some cough medicine, and then the girls got all dramatic about it. They do that, my daughters, since their mum had to go in a home, which is another thing. I wanted to be with Edna, not stuck in a waiting room.

Load of fuss for nothing. I'm 76 years old; just give me the medicine, and I'll get on with it, as I always have. But, oh no, bossy boots, our Diana gets involved, and before I know where I am, it's a family outing.

Harry's story is a typical example of a patient who has no idea what might be the cause of his symptoms, has a family who love him desperately, and may have an idea that this might be bad news. All of them are hopeful, and all of them are relying on clear information and for Harry to be treated kindly by the professionals he is about to meet: the professionals who will assess him. From a clinical perspective, it seems that Harry has lung cancer, inoperable lung cancer, probably with a poor prognosis. For Harry and his family, this is likely to be one of the worst days of their lives.

DOI: 10.1201/9781003427377-4

Preassessment Considerations

First, be prepared! Is all the necessary information available? Is the treatment plan known? Is it reasonable/possible for the patient to have a carer there at the time of assessment, should they wish to? Are there any sensory impairments or language difficulties to take into consideration? Professionals should not begin any communication with the patient before answering the preceding questions and satisfying themselves that they have all the information that they will need. It's part of being professional.

Assessments may take place at the point of diagnosis and at other key points, such as changes in prognosis and the development of symptoms necessitating the need for other services. The skills described in this chapter can be used when assessing a patient at any point in the journey. It is a continual process and should be made by a professional with the appropriate level of skills and knowledge.[3] Any subsequent assessments need to build on previous assessments to reduce duplication and prevent patients from being asked similar questions repeatedly.

Multidisciplinary assessment should only happen when a person consents to the process. Consent must be given before the person's information is shared with, and within, separate organisations, in line with legal requirements and obligations.

The following are useful headings for any assessment and sharing of information:

- Who is this person?
- History of current problem
- Relevant past medical history
- Family issues
- Social issues
- Financial situation
- Psychological aspects
- Summary

First, when meeting a patient for the first time, it is important to think about how best to approach them. Remember the confidence component. Approach with courtesy, warmth, and purpose. Patients have a level of expectation regarding all interactions. Someone who seems to know why they are there and what they are doing and displays a confident, friendly attitude will reassure them. A professional introduction must be clear. Patients have met so many professionals at this point in their journey, and whilst professionals understand all the different titles and responsibilities, patients usually do not. Note: it is worth being honest about possible problems which may need to be considered when meeting a patient for the first time. Information involves more than just words.

JOE'S STORY AND THE IMPACT OF LABELS!

I knew it was bad news. We were taken into an office to see the consultant and there was a nurse there. She was looking kindly at us, and she had a badge which read 'Palliative Care Clinical Nurse Specialist'. I wasn't sure what the badge meant, but I knew that this was different from other appointments and that the news wasn't going to be good, so I reached out for Elizabeth's hand and we braced ourselves.

Strange environments, new professionals, badges, and a different manner and tone all send signals and warning shots to patients and their carers. Communication is much more than words, and chances are, as professionals are introducing themselves, patients and their carers are mentally assimilating the new knowledge and reacting emotionally to it. Human communication is 20% verbal and 80% non-verbal,[4] and reading a badge can be a bad way to find out a diagnosis or prognosis.

There are no hard-and-fast rules here. Professionals are also picking up clues from the patient and processing new knowledge. It may be that such clues are valuable, a 'warning shot', and therefore clinically appropriate. Conversely, it may be that removing a badge for the first assessment is preferable. Consider the message sent out at the first meeting, by having 'Hospice' or 'Macmillan Cancer Relief' written on a badge.

Often when palliative care professionals are involved, it is because another clinician has asked for their input, possibly for support or symptom management advice. The referring clinician, already known to the patient, may introduce the new professional and state her reasons for requesting her input. This can be helpful and may have taken place before the palliative care professional meets the patient. For example, the referring clinician may have said something like, 'I am going to ask one of my colleagues to see you; she will be able to help with your pain or offer more support to you and your wife'. If such reasons have been stated in a previous conversation with the patient, ask the referring clinician about these discussions and read the referral forms carefully. This information should form part of your introduction; it helps to show continuity of care, effective clinical liaison, and good working relationships, all of which help make the patient feel more confident in the system on which they rely. Patients need to know that professionals work well together and stating that you are on the same clinical agenda as the consultant/clinician in whom they have confidence is always helpful. For example, 'My name is Sue, I am one of the specialist nurses working with Dr Brown', and if your instincts suggest that not wearing a badge for the first assessment is the right thing to do, remove it. Follow your instincts; they are there to guide you. The chances are that, after a therapeutic relationship has been formed during the assessment, some fearful myths will have been dispelled, and wearing the badge next time will be okay. Of course, there will be organisational and management rules to think about, but communication has to be about being human, and common sense and kindness are part of that. Whilst, as stated, there are no hard-and-fast rules, sensitivity and caution are important. Theories and models are necessary; that they work in practice is vital. This tension is, in reality, something that experienced professionals balance on a daily basis, without ever acknowledging it.

Sitting down at the start of a consultation (whenever possible) helps create an impression that you have the time to listen (even when your time is finite). For the same reason those working in the community can achieve this by removing their coat (if they are wearing one). The offer of a drink can be refused because you have only just had one, rather than just 'no thank you'. Such small actions relax the patient and their carer by stopping them from feeling rushed and just one of many patients that you are seeing (even though, of course, they are).

Having introduced yourself, it is important to consider how the patient wants to be addressed. Society in general may seem to be less formal, but there remain some patients who prefer to be addressed formally, such as 'Miss Smith', for example. The professional must not impose their own style at the point of introduction; it is easy to discomfort someone immediately by assuming they are happy to be spoken to informally. A quick and clear question to elicit this information helps, such as 'Would you like me to call you Miss Smith or Mildred?'

The Assessment Process: Who Is This Person?

After the introductions, answers to the preceding question will crystallise. There will have been an indication of the preferred style of communication and language to be used. It is possible, for example, that the patient may have used humour to set the tone, offering insights into the type of person they are. It is usually easy to identify anxiety and distress. The people who are important to the patient may be there at the first assessment, and scrutiny of the relationship between them begins. As part of the introduction, it is helpful to ask permission to jot things down. It is respectful and prevents the patient from assuming that the professional is not listening as she writes. All patients understand that documentation is necessary, but when permission is gained, the professional can soften the atmosphere by stating that she will summarise any problems and make a plan at the end of the assessment. It allows the patient to feel comfortable that his concerns are being documented for the purpose of returning to them at the end of the assessment. It's all about confidence, about developing the patient's confidence in the new professional.

All information gathered at the assessment must be documented clearly to facilitate accurate data collection and ensure safe practice within the multi-professional team. These issues are everyone's responsibility and can provide useful insights. For example, an engineer (working or retired) may benefit from a different communication style than, for example, an administrator. The patient's background is informative, and communication styles are often altered in light of this insight. For example, an engineer will generally appreciate very clear, solution-orientated information, with descriptions of the science behind the decision and even diagrams; this encourages compliance with treatment and demonstrates individual care planning.

Eliciting a patient's value system is vital and can be achieved by asking simple and direct questions throughout the assessment, such as 'What is the most important thing to you?' 'Who is the most important person in your life?' 'What is your biggest fear?' and 'Are you someone who likes all the information in detail, or a person who likes to hear things bit by bit?'

Sometime, professionals shy away from such a questioning style as it feels too direct, but that is what patients expect and need. They appreciate a clear and confident approach that gives them the opportunity to tell a professional what is important to them. The information gathered becomes pivotal in the relationship and forms part of the contract between the patient and the professional. If their dog is their biggest worry, acknowledge this.

Patients are not interested in what professionals think. They need to know that professionals are interested in what they, the patient, think.

A patient may or may not have a strong faith; if they do and this isn't acknowledged and fostered, it may be spiritually shattering for the patient. Listen and then communicate understanding.

History of Their Current Problems

A detailed account of a patient's whole medical history isn't always needed although sometimes, patients like to tell it, and this can be time-consuming. The palliative care assessment has to relate to clinically relevant issues and focusing the patient on what is relevant takes a kind firmness and skill. Starting this part of the assessment can be helped by using some simple sentences, for example, 'I have read your notes and am aware of what has happened with your illness so far', or 'Dr Brown has filled me in and I am aware that you have had a difficult time recently'. Then perhaps follow this with 'It would really help me if you could tell me when the problems first started' or 'I was wondering how you were feeling about things?'

At this point, the professional will have judged the type of language used by the patient. Everyone has a different type and level of intelligence and vocabulary available to them. A person lacking in formal education may be highly emotionally intelligent, whilst an academic professor may use long words and speak in a formal style but fail to pick up the subtle messages from those around him. People are fascinating, and getting to know and understand them is such a rewarding process. When possible, it helps if the professional can mirror the language and vocabulary used by the patient. It shows and helps understanding, and patients feel more at ease. What is obviously worrying to the professional may lack significance to the patient. The patient's perspective is crucial: reading the clinical notes is easy, but finding out what the patient thinks the diagnosis means is harder.

Asking the patient when they first noticed something was wrong focuses them on the start of their illness. Knowing what their first symptoms were provides a lot of information. Professionals are experts in pattern recognition, i.e., the details that get them to a diagnosis or decision. For example, professionals recognise unexplained weight loss or bleeding as worrying signs. The date and nature of initial symptoms and investigations must be documented; this will also give relevant information to the next professional who uses the patient's notes. It states what the patient has been through, physically and mentally, and can often give clear prognostic indicators. Discussing symptoms will lead to what happens next and will inform the assessor about other professionals involved in the patient's care.

Typically, the patient will have seen their GP, who may have started treatment, ordered investigations, or referred him to a specialist.

How long it took to get a diagnosis and their feelings related to this may be issues that the patient wants to discuss during the first assessment. It is valuable information for the professional and allows her to understand what the patient has endured so far and for how long and which clinicians are involved in his care.

Knowing which investigations have been done or ordered is vital in order to advise or support a patient. As the professional shows an understanding of this information, the patient's confidence in her will start to grow.

At this stage, the professional can see clearly what has happened so far and which clinician is responsible for the patient's care. The next stage is to ask directly what the patient understands from what has been said so far. Are they expecting bad news or not? Do they fully understand the impact of what has been said? Asking, 'What is your understanding of the situation so far?' is helpful. The answer will inform the professional how best to proceed. It may not be appropriate for the professional to give further information or insight at this time. This is the assessment stage, the time to start a relationship of trust that the patient will need later. A gentle approach using clear questions and documentation is often all that is needed.

Having discovered the level of the patient's understanding, it is important to move on to how the patient feels, both psychologically and physically, and it helps to ask just that: 'How are you feeling about things?' The patient will choose his own priorities and may discuss the physical or psychological aspects. Listening to his priorities is helpful, acknowledging what has been said is vital. For example, 'This has been a very difficult time for you; I will try to help with that'.

If a patient's initial response to any question about feelings is to talk of the physical symptoms, the professional must go with that agenda. The order in which the assessment is completed doesn't matter, but it does matter that the professional is 'in the moment' with the patient. It is their priorities that matter. It is easy to shift the discussion to cover psychological aspects or concerns and expectations later.

As this is a clinical relationship, the professional will need to know which symptoms the patient is experiencing now and, most importantly, which symptoms are bothering them most. When a patient mentions a symptom, further questioning about the nature of the symptom is needed; for example, 'What is the nature of the pain?' 'How long have you had it?' 'When do you get it?' or 'Does anything help or make it worse?' This information will help the professional to understand both how the problem affects the patient and its current management.

Relevant Past Medical History

The patient's past medical history is important; it helps to ask the patient about any serious illnesses. This can help the patient avoid giving a long history of irrelevant illnesses. Often a patient may deny having any other medical problems, but the list of medicines being taken tells another story. The patient's answers to questions about both medical history and current medication are needed to get a full picture.

A list of medicines, for example, may indicate cardiac or respiratory disease, hypertension, or depression. Some medicines may clearly be being taken for prophylactic reasons, such as statins, and some for therapeutic reasons, such as antibiotics.

As people live longer, they acquire more chronic illnesses and therefore see more professionals, any patient will have met dozens of different professionals on his journey. It is therefore easier to get information mixed up and for him not to know what to report to whom when he finds himself in numerous clinical situations.

During the assessment, the professional is building a picture of the patient in her mind. The patient may not deem all the information given to be important, but to a professional, it may be very useful. For example, if the patient is a diabetic, it will affect whether steroids can be used. If he has a history of gastric problems, an anti-inflammatory drug may be contraindicated. Significant information should be highlighted for the benefit of other professionals and as a reminder to the assessing professional. Any known drug allergies need to be carefully documented and explored. If a patient states that he has an allergy, the professional should explore the nature of the reaction. Patients don't know the difference between a side effect and an allergy, and they may have been labelled as allergic unnecessarily. For example, nausea is a common side effect of antibiotics, whereas swelling of the airway is a significant allergic reaction.

Family Issues

Having gathered all the relevant clinical information, the professional can move on to other domains, such as finding out who is important to the patient. This may or may not be family, a fact that gave birth to the term *significant others*. The important questions are,

Who is the person most important to the patient? Who has the patient chosen to care for and support them? and, crucially, Are they happy for professionals to speak to this person should they need to ask questions about the patient's condition? Gaining clarity and documenting this information can make later communication much simpler.

Enquiries about the patient's family should include a detailed and accurate genogram. This will give insight into any possible genetic links or hereditary diseases and what the patient may have already seen and been affected by.

Also, any estrangements between family members can be noted. These can be problematic later on, and it is important to state that the professional can only be responsible for documenting what the patient has told her. Sometimes, there may be family members that the patient chooses not to mention; that is his choice, and that is the only agenda the professional can work with.

Modern families can be complex, with second or third marriages or children from several relationships. The important issue is simple – Who is important to the patient? Drawing a circle around those who live with the patient can be very useful information in terms of assessing care and future needs.

It may be that at this stage of the assessment, the main carer is obvious to the professional. Family dynamics can be very interesting, and there is often a key person within the family who supports the patient and takes most of the responsibility for caregiving. Conversely, family members who live away often worry and may even feel guilty and may therefore ring regularly for updates and information. There may even be a family member who is a healthcare professional.

Rather than dreading this, the professional should consider how this might feel and should communicate with this family member in the manner that they would wish to receive information if they were in the same position. It is possible that this family member expects the professional to dread their input and may overcompensate by communicating less than they would wish to. If it is the patient's wish, this family member should be included in important discussions. They have knowledge that may make their burden greater, and it is likely that the rest of the family is relying on them to have all the answers and to think clearly and make decisions when they also are coping with a difficult situation.

Social Issues

Future care will be tailored to the patient's needs, and these will vary according to the social situation. The type of accommodation, whether it is a flat, house, or bungalow and whether it is owned or rented, all have an impact on future care plans. Eliciting this information can be helpful both for the assessor and for the professionals involved in the patient's future care. If the house is rented, it may not be possible to provide adaptations, meaning stairs may become a problem for the patient as the illness progresses, and as the context of this book is palliative care, the illness will, by definition, progress.

As the assessment is being done in the patient's home, noting that space is available for a bed downstairs or how many steps there are into the property can be useful. This type of information should be written in the patient's notes. It is all written for the patient's benefit; professionals share patient care and therefore need to communicate clearly and effectively.

Family may not be the main carers of the patient; this role may be taken on, or complemented, by friends, neighbours, pastoral services, or members of social groups. Assessing the support available is valuable. Social Services/home care may already be involved. The patient may, in fact, be the main carer for a sick relative, and this can be the cause of much distress. Understanding this and offering support when possible is very helpful. Older people are often caring for a frail partner, and this will affect the decisions they make regarding treatment options and future care. It is not unknown for both members of a relationship to have a life-threatening disease at the same time. Similarly, patients may be the carer for a child with learning difficulties or have learning difficulties themselves.

Every professional has their limitations, and the knowledge of other professionals caring for the patient can be valuable so communication with them (with the patient's consent) is vital.

Financial Issues

Illness can have a devastating effect on the financial stability and psychological well-being of a patient and his family. The patient may be the main, or only, wage earner in the family. The financial resources and sick leave entitlements of patients vary widely and must be carefully assessed. The level of stress caused by such money worries can be huge. People often define themselves partly by the job they do and the role they have within the family. Being too unwell to work can be catastrophic to the patient's psychological well-being, as well as his financial security.

If the assessing professional is able to advise on and apply for benefits, it is important to do so as soon as possible. Fifty per cent of patients dying from cancer receive neither the higher rate of Disability Living Allowance nor Attendance Allowance.[5] It may be the most important outcome of an assessment. It is difficult to think clearly during illness, and benefit forms are notoriously complex, so taking this task off a patient's worry list is greatly appreciated. If the assessing professional doesn't have time or if the patient's financial situation is complex, then referring to a benefits advisor may be preferable. They are experts in this field, but they will appreciate comprehensive details of the patient's situation including unique identifiers, such as their National Insurance number.

Psychological Issues

If the patient hasn't already discussed this by the end of an assessment, it is important that the professional addresses this aspect directly. Changes in body image, financial status, and spiritual and sexual issues will quite possibly have affected his psychological state. Change itself is stressful, and change that adversely affects someone's future can be devastating. Using an open, gentle question helps facilitate this, such as 'I was wondering how you're coping with all this?' or 'Often patients can feel very worried about things; is that the case for you?' Sometimes patients don't realise how they are feeling until they stop and think about it and then verbalise it. This may be the first time they have been asked about their feelings. When patients don't ask questions or state their fears, it is important that the professional doesn't assume that they don't have any. It can quite simply mean that they haven't been given the opportunity to discuss them. Addressing this aspect of care is everyone's responsibility, and it doesn't take long. Finding out how the patient feels and copes now will save time later on.

An assessment is about getting to know the patient and how he functions as a human being. An assessment which doesn't address the psychological issues is incomplete. If the patient offers a cue or a revealing sentence, then documenting this in the notes, in speech marks can be very useful for other professionals involved. For example, 'It's the thought of pain that scares me most'.

Spiritual concerns are distinct from religious beliefs; they relate to how a person defines themselves and whether they see their life as having meaning. Asking the patient whether he has a faith that is important to him will elicit a clear response regarding religious values, which must be respected and provided for, if possible. The crucial aspect of assessing a patient's psychological needs is to ascertain clearly what his value system is, and asking the right questions to elicit this information is an acquired skill.

The patient may quite clearly say what kind of person he is, whether he is someone who wants to stay positive for as long as possible and not discuss such issues as 'how long' or, conversely, someone who wants all the information in detail and regularly. Such clear statements are made for a reason, possibly reasons that the professional can't immediately understand, but they should be noted and respected, because they translate to 'This is how I am coping at the moment'. Everyone will choose their own strategy for coping, and it will inevitably change throughout the journey, for both patients and carers, which is why assessments need to be made and remade at key points.

If the patient has not made his preferred style of communication clear, it is sensible and respectful to ask at this point. Using a friendly, simple question can help, such as 'Everyone is different, some people prefer to have information when they need to know it and stay positive, and some like lots of information in detail. It would help me to know which kind of person you are'.

Patients don't mind answering this; in fact, they gain a sense of control here and consequently feel safer in psychological terms.

Having carried out and clearly documented a holistic assessment, it is crucial that the professional asks the patient what his biggest concern is. This may be a completely different concern from those identified by the professional during the assessment. It is vital to deal effectively with both, if possible.

If the problem is one that the professional can't help with herself, then referral to someone who can is needed, and if it is a problem that can't actually be solved, the professional should be explicit about this. Sometimes the most honest answer is 'I don't know'. Professionals should not pressure themselves to feel that they must always have all the answers. It isn't possible, but fortunately, given the nature of healthcare, it is usually possible to identify another professional who does know.

Summary

A summary is an opportunity for the professional to show that she has heard the patient, not just listened but heard, and that she has registered his worries and priorities, outlined the plan for dealing with those problems, and made a contract of how the patient–professional relationship will be. This should reflect the patient's preferred communication style and outline the professional's role and future availability.

MARY'S STORY

Tony, thank you for sharing all that with me and for letting me scribble away while you were talking. This has obviously been a very difficult time for you and it has really helped me to understand how you feel.

You tell me you are a man who likes straight talking, and I promise to give you clear honest information at all times. From what you tell me, your biggest concerns at the moment are nausea and money issues. I am going to chat with your doctor about changing your anti-sickness medicine and get the necessary benefit forms completed and sent off for you. I think that is the most useful thing I can do today. My role as a specialist nurse means that I am only involved when you have more complex problems relating to your illness. Your GP and community nurse will continue to be your key people and regular callers. If it is okay with you, I would like to see you again in a few days to check on how you are coping with your new medicine. I have written down what we have agreed today and put my contact details there, should you or your family want to speak to me. I am available during office hours, and if you leave me a message, I will return your call as soon as possible. Are there any further questions? Is there anything else I can help you with today? If you think of anything do ring me; you have taken in a lot of information today and you might think of something later. Is that okay with you? I will look forward to seeing you in a few days and please do contact me if you want to.

Mary's story illustrates many valuable points. She has reflected back Tony's main concerns, showing that she has heard and understood; she has reassured him of her professional plan and made her role clear to avoid Tony having unrealistic expectations of her. Her promise to respect Tony's need for honest information is very important; it helped build trust from the outset. Tony will also now understand the roles of those involved in his care and accept the communication between them. He will know who his key worker is and has written information should he forget the agreed plan from the assessment. Patients with a life-threatening illness often feel that there is nothing more that can be done. Mary has demonstrated in a professional manner that there is, and she is doing it.

There is an art to forming relationships and behaving in a confident manner, which also demonstrates kindness and warmth. Gentleness is the greatest of all strengths.

Listening well, picking up and responding to cues is an art. Professionals see, hear, listen, and show that they have understood. It's not a simple task; it's complex and expert practitioners do it every day. Often, they make it look easy; that is what experts do. There is a saying 'If it looks hard work, then you are not working hard enough'. Professionals do work hard. To be with a patient throughout their illness is very hard. If they get the first assessment right, then the patient will choose to come back to them when they need to. No professional can be omnipresent; often they have to rely on the patient contacting them when help is needed. If a professional uses the science and art of the skills outlined in this chapter, from diagnosis to death, the patient, and those who love them, will benefit.

A difficult situation will have been made easier to bear, and in the absence of curative treatment, that is the greatest reward for palliative care professionals.

TIP: *The reason we have two ears and one mouth is that we may listen more and talk less.*

References

1. Saunders C. The treatment of intractable pain in terminal cancer. *Proc Roy Soc Med*. 1963; **56**: 195–197.
2. World Health Organization. *Cancer Pain Relief*. Geneva: WHO; 1996.
3. National Institute of Clinical Excellence. *Improving Supportive and Palliative Care for Adults with Cancer*. London: NICE; 2004.
4. Mehrabian A. *Silent Messages*. Belmont, CA: Wadsworth; 1971.
5. Macmillan Cancer Support. *Unclaimed millions*. Available at: http://www.macmillan.org.uk/Aboutus/News/Latest_News/CancerPatientsLoseOutOnMillionsOfUnclaimedBenefits.aspx (2009; accessed June 2011).

5

Diagnosis

How would it feel to be forced to join a club that you don't want to join?

Clinical Language

For clinicians who work and function in clinical arenas, it is important both to use and be prepared to explain clinical language. This is vital if the patient is to understand from the beginning what is happening to them. When discussing cancer, remember that it is a diagnosis. Emotive phrases such as 'a battle' or 'a war' do not help patients and are therefore best left with the journalists, whose sole aim is to sell newspapers. Oft-used euphemisms have largely been relegated to the archives of medical language; their time has gone, in the face of open discussion, increased patient choice and the need for patient consent to treatment. Cancer is not the big 'C'; neither is it 'ca'; it's 'cancer'. It is not a polyp and not just a growth; it is a type of tumour: the malignant type. It is vital that professionals use clear language to patients and unambiguous terms. 'Wishy-washy' terms do not aid understanding and receiving a diagnosis of a life-threatening disease is hard enough without the water being muddied by using more palatable, saccharine phrases. This isn't meant to sound dictatorial; it is just so important that professionals are just that – professional; it's what the patient needs. They have friends and lay carers who will attempt to soften the blow with such language, but in order to support the patient well and right from the beginning, professionals have to be professional in their communication style.

The Staging Process

By the time of diagnosis, patients will have endured various and sometimes unpleasant investigations. If the diagnosis is cancer, they may, or may not, have been through the complicated staging process. It is important to acknowledge from the beginning that uncertainty itself can be distressing. The staging process, as the name suggests, is done to determine the site, type, and stage of the cancer. In terms of oncology treatments, this process is very important because it enables oncologists to prescribe and monitor the most effective treatments. Staging may have included some, or all, of the following: X-rays and other scans, blood tests, and surgical resection biopsies. Other factors, including the patient's general health and his preferences, as well as various biochemical tests on cancer

DOI: 10.1201/9781003427377-5

cells will contribute to determining the prognosis and treatment. So, while the stage is important, it is not everything.

It is not uncommon for the site and type of a primary tumour to remain unidentified, being recorded as an unknown primary (UKP). Up to 30% of all cancers are UKPs. This can be both upsetting and very difficult for patients to understand. The news that the primary cancer can't be identified often provokes patients to use a sentence beginning with 'In this day and age ...'. A cancer cell is, by definition, a mutated cell and therefore can be difficult to identify. It can also be difficult to see in radiological investigations. This may well be something that the professional will have to be prepared to explain. Medicine, despite many technological advances, still does not have all the answers that patients want. A clear diagnosis for many diseases is not always possible. In those circumstances, doctors working in all specialties offer the best advice and treatment that they can.

There is an argument against blunt diagnostic labelling; it can seem too harsh when given early in the process. It is important that the professional explores the patient's experience of the disease which has been diagnosed. A family member or friend quite possibly had a similar condition, and unless they are addressed, unnecessary fears can form early on. The patient's experience may have been negative, and misperceptions and misinterpretations can form quickly and may relate to situations that don't and/or won't apply, such as hair loss, dementia, or paralysis.

Information Network

At the time of diagnosis, it helps to advise the patient and his carers against searching the internet for terms that don't apply. This adds weight to the importance of giving clear information at the outset. Patients tend not to state their intention to do this, but often appear at the next consultation with documents relating to a completely different disease, often from internet sites which are not credible. For example, a patient who has been told that she has breast cancer which has spread to the lymph nodes would not be helped by searching lymph node cancer and applying the information, that will, in fact, relate to lymphoma, not to her own situation. Self-reliance should, of course, be encouraged where it is helpful, and there are many well-researched sites that professionals can recommend. It is appropriate that professionals support patients in making their own choices and utilising helpful information networks.

Diagnosis and Reactions

There are key points in the patient's journey when assessment of his communication needs will be vital. The key points are at diagnosis, at the start and completion of treatment, at each episode of disease recurrence, at the point of recognition of incurability, and at the diagnosis of dying and the start of end-of-life care.

At each of these stages, the professional must negotiate the appropriate level and type of communication needed. This may change as the disease progresses, and the needs of the patient and his carers may not always be compatible. It is always the patient's agenda that should be the primary concern of the professional; the anxieties of others should be noted and addressed separately. This potential conflict in communication needs is discussed in more detail later.

Consultations can be very anxiety-provoking and will follow an already uncertain and often difficult time due to the investigative process. Hearing the diagnosis can be something of a relief to many patients; they may feel it helps to know what they are dealing with and having a name for it may make them feel more empowered to cope. Conversely, it may confirm their worst fears because often, the diagnosis is bad news, which is defined as '[a]ny news that drastically and negatively alters the patient's view of her or his future'.[1]

In a single sentence, the patient's and his carer's lives can change, forever. Suddenly they live in a different world, one where serious disease threatens. They have joined a club that no one wants to join. Few patients are wise about cancer before the event or have read enough about the neurological disease with which they have just been diagnosed. That knowledge belongs to the professional, who will serve the patient well by sitting quietly while the information that has just been given is digested by the family and their carers. During this silence, the patient and his carers are starting the adjustment process, internalising what has been said to them and beginning to form questions in their minds. They may be so shocked that anything that is said afterwards isn't heard at all. Some people 'shut down' at hearing the diagnosis. Recognising this and allowing that silence to last as long as it takes is good practice. It takes skill to remain quiet at such a difficult time, but it is a very important phase for the patient, and the questions that he may ask next or the feelings he verbalises will be very informative for the professional supporting him. The range of normal reactions is vast. Every patient is different: some will respond very pragmatically, and some with strong emotion. The role of the professional is always the same: to assess the patient's communication needs and preferred style, to offer clear information in a kind manner and to write relevant information down for the patient to take away.

Dual Diagnosis

Sadly, the new diagnosis may not be the only illness the patient has. Dual diagnosis and co-morbidities are common. For example, a patient with multiple sclerosis can still develop breast cancer.

KEN'S STORY

I am the carer for my wife who has chronic multiple sclerosis (MS). We have recently been informed that she now has breast cancer and advised that, without chemotherapy, her life expectancy is short. During the last 9 years, I have learnt how to do MS, but I have no idea how to do breast cancer. There is no preparation for disability, and suddenly when you think it can't get any worse, it gets a lot worse; she has breast cancer.

How do you tell someone who has been to hell and back that they have to go again? She told me that the worst part of having MS was not so much losing control, as having no control over it. No cure, no treatment given and no choice. She is more afraid of MS than she is of breast cancer. 'I can control what is wrong with my breast; I can have it cut off' was how she decided to cope with the news. So, you put it behind you, but you wish you had never read *Before I Say Goodbye*, and you daren't even think of what will happen next. I used to believe that knowledge is power, which is to say that I can handle things better if I know what the next stage of illness will be. Now, it only serves to fuel the fear in me. As far as this cancer is concerned, I want knowledge to be dispensed on a need-to-know basis. In my case, less is better right now.

Ken's story describes well just how catastrophic a diagnosis can be, that professionals can never assume that the illness being diagnosed is the only illness the patient has or the only source of stress for him and his carers. Fate can be so unkind to people, and professionals can be shocked by the amount of trauma one person and his carers can have to cope with.

The experiences, feelings, and fears of patients and their carers will vary enormously, but the priorities and purpose of the professional that have been outlined must never change. A useful maxim is 'the more complex a situation is, the more important it is to stick to the basic rules'. It is easy to become overwhelmed with the magnitude of problems that patients and their carers face, but the professional must stay on solid ground when the ground beneath others is shaking. Ken quite clearly tells us that for the moment, he only wants to hear what he needs to know at this time. He is understandably overwhelmed and is stating the level of communication that he needs at the present time. His wish can therefore be acknowledged, understood, and respected. He has highlighted that his communication needs have changed and demonstrated that he is, and no doubt will continue to be, clear about this. Ken has made it easy for the professional to assess and support him. His story of how the diagnosis has affected him is truly illuminating.

Patients will often have both short- and long-term fears, for example: 'Will I have to have time off work? 'No, I don't want to go the way Paul did; it was horrendous at the end'. Their immediate responses must be noted by the professional and dealt with during the summary at the end of the consultation.

The Right Support

It is helpful to the patient if the diagnosis is given by the doctor who made it and is responsible for the patient's care, as it is likely that the patient and/or his carers will have questions that the diagnosing doctor will be best placed to answer. Other professionals play a valuable role in this process and may be the best people to explain further about the diagnosis and what was discussed during the consultation. When patients and their carers are struggling to think straight, the clear and gentle support of other professionals is greatly appreciated. Many helpful leaflets can be given to patients and their carers at the point of diagnosis, leaflets that explain the disease; the treatment, if appropriate; and the services available. This information can be taken away and read at a later date.

As long as they have the appropriate skills and knowledge to meet the patient's needs, any professional involved in his care can undertake subsequent discussions relating to his case. There are no laws that state that all clinical discussion has to be with a doctor. Patients and their carers will identify the professional with whom they feel most comfortable, and it is often that professional, whatever their role, who takes the lead in subsequent discussions. Everyone gravitates to the person with whom they feel the safest and most comfortable at times of crisis and illness is no different. Professional parochialism is divisive to care and in conflict with the ethos of multidisciplinary practice of modern healthcare. No single professional 'owns' the patient, and no professional can function without the support of others. Communication with relevant colleagues is therefore crucial, absolutely crucial.

If the diagnosis has been given in the outpatient hospital setting, the patient's GP and community nurse should be informed as soon as possible. If the patient is currently an inpatient in the hospital, then the ward team of doctors and nurses should be informed. They are the key workers for the patient.

Specialists dip in and out of care when the patient has specialist problems. Whilst they are specialists, they are not special, and it is often the key workers who carry out most of the care and know the patient best. At such a difficult time, patients and their carers may need an increased level of support, and understanding and providing the key workers with up-to-date and clear information, in both verbal and written forms, enables the network of support to be effectively placed around the patient and his carers. Key workers cannot possibly support the patient without the necessary information. It is irrelevant who meets the patient's needs as long as someone does. If care is to be seamless, which is definitely the most effective type of care, then information must follow the patient, and it is everyone's responsibility to make sure that this happens. Professionals work extremely hard to achieve this and upgraded and newly designed information technology is making it easier, but often a quick phone call to the relevant professional is the best way to relay important information. It is crucial to pass information to the appropriate people and valuable to not share it with those professionals who *don't* need to know. A professional's time is often wasted listening to information relating to patients who are *not* in their care. As all professionals are extremely busy, providing information that is not relevant to their workload is unhelpful and time-consuming.

The following 5-point checklist is useful:

- Am I addressing the right person? (Does this professional know the patient well?) Have I asked the professional whom I think I should contact?
- What do I know about this patient that the other professional should know? What do I need to know from the other professional?
- What does this mean for the patient's future care?
- Who is going to do what? Who is now responsible for the care of this patient?
- How shall we communicate in the future?

Much communication is impeded because professionals don't want to step on each other's toes!

The diagnosis may explain and make sense of the symptoms that the patient has been experiencing. This can be reassuring for the patient; often he has been considering himself weak and berating himself for not being able to fight the symptoms off. Carers also may suddenly understand why, for example, the patient's appetite has diminished so much or

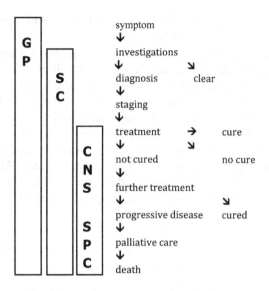

FIGURE 1
The patient's journey involving the general practitioner (GP), specialist care (SC, whether non-malignant diseases or oncology, including surgeons), and a clinical nurse specialist in specialist palliative care (CNS SPC).

why his mood has altered so dramatically. Current symptoms must be noted, and past and current treatment should form part of the clinical summary.

In any situation in palliative care, it is vital that professionals concentrate on what can be done. Even when no curative treatment is possible, there is always something that can be done and said to help the situation. Palliative care, by definition, means to relieve the bad effects of something. Concentrating on what can be done to help can make a huge difference in how people cope. There are occasions when the outcome/prognosis is genuinely unknown; cure may or may not be achievable. However, it is still appropriate for palliative care professionals to be involved in the early stages. Conversely, the diagnosis may also carry a very poor prognosis, which entails telling the patient that his life expectancy is very short. This is traumatic and usually shocking information for the patient and his carers. It is definitely a consultation which includes breaking bad news and requires the necessary skills for this. These skills are discussed in more detail later. The flow chart in Figure 1 illustrates the need for palliative care input throughout a patient's typical cancer journey.

This flow chart also indicates that patients and their carers will meet many different professionals during their illness. Making new relationships and understanding the various roles can be very taxing for patients; constant summarising and the offer of written information are always useful.

The Level of Hope

It is appropriate to assume that patients will have been hoping for good news at the point of diagnosis: hoping that it wasn't serious, that it wasn't the disease they most dreaded. Hope is a fluid concept within healthcare. It will change, from hoping that their initial fears are not realised to hoping that there is something that can be done, that the treatment will work, that the disease will not recur, that their symptoms can be controlled to hoping for quality of life, which includes a peaceful death.

A patient's changing level of hope must be noticed and acted upon by professionals. Often, hope is a sustaining factor, and to remove it entirely would be very damaging to how the patient is coping at that time. It is entirely reasonable for the patient to hope that any treatment prescribed will be helpful. That is, after all, the clinical objective. However, inappropriate hope must be carefully challenged. For example, allowing a patient to book a holiday for the next year when the professional knows that, even with treatment, he is unlikely to be well enough, isn't helpful. Whilst professionals don't have all the answers, they do have more experience and knowledge than the patient and it is important that they use it. Advising that they put off making big decisions at the moment may be enough. Patients are usually happy to take advice and giving the best advice is sometimes the most useful action a professional can take.

ANDREW'S STORY

Mary's daughter, Paula, seemed so angry at the diagnosis. She was challenging the consultant and disagreeing with the poor prognosis that Mary had been given, clearly because she couldn't cope with the pain of facing the news. Mary was very frail and jaundiced, not medically fit enough for treatment, struggling to stay awake and trying so hard to sound grateful to her daughter when Paula promised she would book the African safari that Mary had always dreamed of. I could see that Mary hadn't the heart or strength to tell her that she didn't want to think about it. Paula was adamant, and she was going home to book it. I pointed out how much care her mum would need in the coming weeks. 'We will wing it' was her reply, and she was clearly annoyed with me.

I had to draw breath and choose my words carefully, for both their sakes. 'I know that this is hard for you to accept, but it is my job to give you the best advice. I wouldn't be helping you if I didn't. I'm so sorry, Paula, but Mum is not fit to travel abroad. You will not be able to get the necessary medical insurance. She will become very unwell, and the services you will both need won't be there. The result will be catastrophic for you both. The lovely memories you want to make won't happen. It will become a stressful nightmare for you both'. I paused to allow my words to sink in.

'I can see how much you love your mum and I know that that is the last thing you would want to happen. I think it would be better if you had a chat when you got home, when you have both had time to rest and think, and then perhaps she will be able to tell you if there is something special she would like to do, something that is easier for her. There may be something lovely and close to home that she would really enjoy, and we would be able to help you with that. I'm sorry, this is disappointing for you, but I have to try to keep Mum safe and give you good advice'.

Mary looked so relieved, and it was hard to watch the reality dawn on Paula; she looked so defeated by my words, but on reflection, I know I had chosen my words well and offered the best advice possible, with kindness as my main intention and because of my many years of experience, and I know, from that experience, that I can't improve on that.

Andrew is honest with us that it has taken many years of experience for him to be brave enough to challenge inappropriate hope well. He has learnt that he is not the patient's friend or lay carer; he is the professional, with responsibilities, who knows more about the illness than the patient and their carer, and he has been brave enough to use that knowledge to help both the patient and her loving daughter.

Pressure

Having been fully informed of the diagnosis, it is common for the patient and/or his carers to ask about treatment options. The question may even be followed by a phrase such as 'I am in your hands, Doc'. It helps the doctor-to-patient relationship if such phrases are challenged from the outset. Whilst all clinicians will do their utmost to help the patient in every way, accepting such a level of responsibility can be an unhelpful pressure. Palliative care is about disease that can't be cured. The meaning of the term *palliation* should always be in a professional's mind. Emotive statements like 'I am in your hands, Doc' and 'I couldn't cope without you' may be ego-boosting but may foster inappropriate expectations and an unhelpful dependent relationship which ultimately will not help the patient at all. Patients do cope when professionals aren't there; they have to, and they do. They access other people for support, and support cannot always come from one professional.

Understanding Support Systems

It is helpful for the patient to identify a variety of support systems and coping strategies, rather than relying on one particular professional. An outline of the various support systems is therefore very helpful. The different services and roles will have to be explained. Few members of the public could, for example, describe the difference between a Marie Curie nurse and a Macmillan nurse or know that the former has a 'hands-on' nurse at home role and that the latter has a specialist consultative role.

Services have been enhanced by the advent of the site-specific nurse, such as the breast cancer nurse and the lung cancer nurse. However, the roles of the various specialist nurses may be confusing for the patients. Both the site-specific nurse and the palliative care nurse may have their post sponsored by the charity Macmillan Cancer Support and therefore carry the Macmillan title, but they will be working collaboratively, performing different roles according to their different knowledge bases. Specialist nurses are not necessarily sponsored by the Macmillan charity; they may be employed by the National Health Service or by the local hospice. It is important to credit the work of other organisations such as, for example, the British Heart Foundation and motor neurone disease charities, to name but two, for the vital work they carry out in patient care. Not all patients diagnosed with a life-threatening disease have cancer. The work done in the voluntary sector deserves all the praise and respect possible and, in the opinion of the author, a more generous approach to funding.

Macmillan has become synonymous with palliative care, but they sponsor many professionals in many clinical areas; they do not employ or pay ongoing wages. Macmillan sponsorship provides funding for the first 3 years of the professional's post. Macmillan has worked hard to establish its profile and reputation. It has been argued that the public's perception of Macmillan professionals is unrealistic due to the nature of their advertising and professionals will have to dispel such myths and ensure that the patients and their families have understood their role and capabilities. Discussions at the point of diagnosis are very useful, to set the agenda, make agreements, and for professionals to explain how they work. If they are not the key worker, then stating this and adding that they will only visit when there is a problem will help stop the patient from being disappointed later on. Advertising can give the impression that specialist professionals will visit daily or call in just to see if they are needed. In reality, staffing levels are always an issue, and professionals work within their remits and do not make calls purely for social reasons. Patients are very accepting of this when given clear information. All relevant information can be summarised. It is important to repeat the salient facts, which are

- what the patient has been told during the assessment.
- what will happen next, including appointments and investigations.
- discuss and plan changes to the patient's medicines if needed to relieve current symptoms. Communicate with other relevant professionals.
- contact information for the professional with details of availability for the patient and his carers, if the patient consents to this.
- identification of anything the patient doesn't fully understand and offering time to answer any questions that the patient or his carer may have.

The patient and his carers will have been given a lot of information during the process of reaching a diagnosis. It will take time for them to internalise this information and begin the adjustment process. People's responses can be surprising. Everybody is different and professionals support all kinds of people. From diagnosis onwards, professionals are dedicated enough to get to know and support all of them. Understanding what will happen next is crucial, and it can be surprising how many patients have not understood this during the diagnosis consultation. Whatever the prognosis, there will be other consultations, and there will be some sort of treatment.

TIP: Patients are not protected by their ignorance; rather, they are isolated.

Reference

1. Kaye P. *Breaking Bad News*. Northampton: EPL Publications; 1996.

6

Treatment

So, you've told me what I have; what can be done about it?

It's a reasonable question. It would be the first question in everyone's mind. The public (mostly) believes that doctors can cure most diseases 'these days'. However, the harsh reality is that they can cure few diseases, in fact, only two diseases: some infections and some cancers. All other diseases (bear in mind that a broken bone isn't a disease) are either managed/treated, for example, heart disease, bronchitis, arthritis, and diabetes, or they are self-limiting, such as viral infections. Remember that the context of this book is palliative care; acute medicine is not being discussed here.

In terms of life-threatening illnesses, degenerative neurological diseases can only be managed, never cured. Some cancers, depending on their type and stage, can be, and are, cured; some are managed palliatively. Sadly, there are those for which there is no helpful treatment at all, and the best supportive care is the only prescription. Best supportive care can be defined as 'treatment given to prevent, control, or relieve complications and side-effects and to improve the patient's comfort and quality of life'.

Cancer is routinely seen as a terminal condition with excellent palliative care services being involved with the treatment plans. However, a number of life-limiting non-malignant conditions, such as heart failure and chronic obstructive airway disease, just to name two, have mortality rates and a symptom burden comparable to a cancer. Introducing the patient to a palliative care specialist early in the relationship is always helpful.

For this cohort of patients, the journey may be long, there will be numerous admissions to hospital for the symptoms to be stabilised and for symptom control. They will know and trust their treating clinicians greatly, and after being resuscitated from crisis points so many times, it can be hard for both the patient and their family to accept the final phase when it does come.

Repeating the words that 'this cannot be cured' during consultations does help, but adding, 'and we know that you will die eventually from this' helps more to reduce the shock when their body does become overwhelmed. Often a patient may accept that it can't be cured but still not expect death at some time; they often think they will carry on living with a non-curable disease for longer than is realistic.

Such conversations are difficult when the patient has relied on their teams for so long and has been in and out of hospital so often in the past. It is a kindness on the clinician's part to prepare them for the inevitable; for example, heart failure is just that – their heart will eventually fail, and they will eventually die from chronic constructive airway disease.

Within the UK, the diagnosis of cancer and its staging and subsequent treatment options are discussed at a multidisciplinary team meeting (MDT). These meetings are attended by all the clinicians, doctors, and nurses who are relevant to the patient's case. It is where decisions are made, where clinicians share knowledge and expertise, and where each case is carefully discussed allowing all clinicians to offer their opinions and useful information

DOI: 10.1201/9781003427377-6

and to challenge decisions when required. No clinician works in isolation – they are each a spoke in a vast wheel. Modern-day healthcare is about transparency and open discussion; it has moved away from the old-fashioned hierarchy of medical consultants making all the decisions alone. All aspects of the patient's care and all factors affecting treatment decisions are considered. It is a good example of healthcare communication at its best: professionals having open discussions, making joint decisions which keep the patient at the heart of care, recording these decisions accurately and promptly and, crucially, communicating the decisions to all relevant professionals. MDT decisions are carefully recorded, and the patient's own doctor/GP is informed of the decision and the plan. This will include the treatment plan, who is responsible for the treatment and, more importantly, who is responsible for discussing this with the patient, and when. In concise terms, the MDT will record the investigations, staging, diagnosis, treatment plan, and actions to be taken and by whom. This will include which clinician will be responsible for discussing these decisions with the patient. This may be a doctor, nurse or other professional. However, it is reasonable for the doctor, as the prescribing clinician, to be the professional who answers any questions relating to any prescribed treatment and its possible outcomes.

Treatment Types

The three most common treatments for cancer include surgery, chemotherapy, and radiotherapy. Other treatments may include hormonal therapies, biological therapies, laser, or targeted therapy. Treating other life-threatening diseases includes both disease-modifying treatment and drugs to manage symptoms. Supportive care uses various medicines that may improve the quality of life, slow down the disease, or minimise symptoms.

Treatment Aims

Treatment can be given with the aim of curing the disease, controlling it, or relieving symptoms. People are often given more than one type of treatment for their disease.

Cancer Treatments

Surgery

Surgery can be used to diagnose, treat, or even help prevent cancer in some cases. Most people with cancer will have some type of surgery, whether it is diagnostic, curative or reconstructive. Surgery often offers the greatest chance for a cure, especially if the cancer has not spread to other parts of the body.

Cancer testing and treatments improve continually, advances include quicker treatments by injection, more precise oncology treatments, the study of DNA in relation to the development of cancers, more accurate predictions for cancers and the use of artificial intelligence and machine learning may be seen in the future. It is the three main cancer treatments which are discussed here.

Chemotherapy

There are over 50 different chemotherapy drugs that may be used alone or in combination. Different drugs cause different side effects and may be given in a variety of ways.

Chemotherapy Terms

Chemotherapy encompasses a wide variety of therapy treatments. Terms such as *adjuvant*, *neo-adjuvant*, *consolidation*, and *palliative* often add to the confusion surrounding chemotherapy if not properly defined and explained. The purpose of the following list is to explain the various chemotherapy protocols currently used:

- *Adjuvant chemotherapy*. Chemotherapy given to destroy left-over (microscopic) cells that may be present after the known tumour is removed by surgery. Adjuvant chemotherapy is given to prevent a possible cancer recurrence.
- *Neo-adjuvant chemotherapy*. Chemotherapy given prior to the surgical procedure. Neo-adjuvant chemotherapy may be given in an attempt to shrink the cancer so that the surgical procedure may not need to be so extensive.
- *Induction chemotherapy*. Chemotherapy given to induce remission. This term is commonly used in the treatment of acute leukaemias.
- *Consolidation chemotherapy*. Chemotherapy given once a remission is achieved. The goal of this therapy is to sustain remission. May also be called intensification therapy. This term is commonly used in the treatment of acute leukaemias.
- *Maintenance chemotherapy*. Chemotherapy given in lower doses to assist in prolonging remission. Maintenance chemotherapy is used only for certain types of cancer, most commonly acute lymphocytic leukaemias and acute promyelocytic leukaemias.
- *First-line chemotherapy*. Chemotherapy that has, through research studies and clinical trials, been determined to have the best probability of treating a given cancer. This may also be called standard therapy.
- *Second-line chemotherapy*. Chemotherapy that is given if a disease has not responded or has recurred after first-line chemotherapy. Second-line chemotherapy, through research studies and clinical trials, has been determined to be effective in treating a given cancer that has not responded or recurred after standard chemotherapy. In some cases, this may also be referred to as salvage therapy.
- *Palliative chemotherapy*. Palliative chemotherapy is given specifically to address symptom management without expecting to significantly reduce the cancer.

Cancer Trials

What Are Cancer Clinical Trials?

In the discussion of cancer treatment, the term *cancer clinical trials* appears frequently. Also called research studies, cancer clinical trials test many types of treatment such as new drugs, new approaches to surgery or radiation therapy and new combinations of treatments. Cancer clinical trials are the first step in testing a new treatment in humans and their goal is to find better ways to treat cancer.

Cancer clinical trials include four different research phases. Each phase answers different questions about the new treatment.

Cancer Clinical Trials: Phase I

The questions being explored in phase I cancer clinical trials are as follows:

- What is the best way to give a new treatment?
- Can this medication be given safely to humans?
- What is a safe dose?

These cancer clinical trials involve a limited number of patients who may not be helped by other known treatments.

Cancer Clinical Trials: Phase II

In phase II of cancer clinical trials, the focus is on learning whether the new treatment has an anticancer effect on a specific cancer. Additional information regarding the side effects of the treatment is also obtained. A small number of people are included because of the risks and unknowns involved.

Cancer Clinical Trials: Phase III

In phase III of cancer clinical trials, the results of people taking a new treatment are compared with the results of people taking a standard treatment. Some of the questions asked in a phase III trial include the following:

- Which group has better survival rates?
- Which group has fewer side effects?

People are assigned at random (a process similar to flipping a coin) to either the new treatment (treatment group) or the current standard treatment (control group). Randomisation helps avoid bias (having the study's results affected by human choices or other factors not related to the treatments being tested). Some cancer clinical trials compare a new treatment with a placebo (a lookalike pill/infusion that contains no active drug). However, a person is told if this is a possibility before deciding whether to take part in a study. Comparing similar groups of people taking a different treatment for the same type of cancer is another way to make sure that the study results are real and caused by the treatment rather than by chance or other factors. These cancer clinical trials may include hundreds to thousands of people from different centres around the country.

Cancer Clinical Trials: Phase IV

In phase IV of cancer clinical trials, also called post-marketing studies, trials are conducted after a treatment has been approved. The purpose of this is to provide an opportunity to learn more details about the treatment, such as

- the mechanism of action,
- fine points regarding toxicities, and
- fine points regarding quality of life,
- questions that may have come up during other phases of cancer clinical trials.

These 'post-marketing' trials may be conducted in a phase I, II, or III format.

What Happens in Cancer Clinical Trials?

In cancer clinical trials, patients receive treatment and doctors carry out research on how the treatment affects patients. A patient's progress is closely monitored during the clinical trial. Once the treatment portion of the clinical trial has been completed, patients may continue to be followed in order to gather information regarding specific endpoints. These endpoints are defined prior to the study being started and may include time to disease progression and/or overall survival.

While cancer clinical trials have risks for the people who take part, each study also takes steps to protect patients. *Cancer clinical trials are often the best treatment approach available.*

Radiotherapy

Radiotherapy is the use of high-energy radiation to destroy cancer cells. It may be used to cure some cancers, to reduce the chance of recurrence or for symptom relief.

About 4 out of 10 people with cancer (40%) have radiotherapy as part of their treatment. It can be given in various ways:

- from outside the body as external radiotherapy using X-rays, 'cobalt irradiation', electrons, and, more rarely, other particles such as protons, and
- from within the body as internal radiotherapy by drinking a liquid that is taken up by cancer cells or by putting radioactive material in, or close to, the tumour.

Biological Therapies

Biological therapies are treatments that use natural substances from the body or drugs made from these substances. They include monoclonal antibodies, cancer growth inhibitors, vaccines and gene therapy. Biological therapies stimulate the body to

- attack or control the growth of cancer cells and
- overcome side effects caused by other cancer treatments such as chemotherapy.

Biological therapies work in a slightly different way to other treatments that kill or control cancer cells. They use a natural substance, or something developed from a natural body substance, to interfere with the way cells interact and signal to each other.

Hormonal Therapies

Hormone treatments use the sex hormones produced in the body or drugs that block them to treat cancer. Not all cancers respond to hormone therapy. Doctors might use hormone therapy for people with cancers that are 'hormone-sensitive' or 'hormone-dependent'. This means that the cancer needs the hormone to grow. Cancers that can be hormone-sensitive are breast cancer, prostate cancer, and womb cancer.

How Hormone Therapy Works

Cancers that are hormone-sensitive or hormone-dependent need hormones to grow. So stopping the hormone from reaching the cancer cells may either slow down or stop the growth of the cancer. Hormone therapies can work by either stopping hormones from being made or preventing the hormone from reaching the cancer cell.

Other Cancer Treatments

Other cancer treatments that might be used are hyperbaric oxygen therapy, photodynamic therapy (PDT), and radiofrequency ablation.

Supportive Therapies

Supportive therapies can be given in addition to or as part of a patient's principal treatment. They include steroids, blood or platelet transfusions, and bisphosphonates.

Treatment with Curative Intent

Having been given a devastating diagnosis of cancer, this is surely the treatment category that everyone would wish to be eligible for. Despite the likely need for further testing/staging and invasive treatment, there is real optimism here; no guaranteed outcomes but real optimism. The prescribing clinician will often discuss relevant research findings.

CASE STUDY – KEEPING LANGUAGE SIMPLE

Patient: 'Oh no! That's awful!'
Doctor: 'The risk of you dying of your cancer is 37%. The treatment can reduce the odds of death by 23%. This represents an absolute reduction in mortality of 8.9% which leads to a progression-free survival rate of 71.4%'.

It's hard for patients to understand the scientific dialogue used, especially if it is couched in medical jargon. Patients and their carers are trying to think straight, to make very important decisions, when often the ground beneath them is shaking. What they need is clear information, guidance, and professional recommendations. It is not too much to expect. No one would expect to make their own decisions on their broken car and its repair; mechanics would give advice, because they know more about cars and how they work. Of course, it would be the customer's decision that the work is done, but helpful advice from a professional who understands the situation better is expected. It should be the same in healthcare. Whilst professionals must ensure that it is the patient's choice to accept a particular prescription offered, it is only fair to share relevant knowledge to support his choices. Professional recommendation is part of the professional's responsibility. Professionals don't know everything, they don't have all the answers, but they know more than the patient, and for that reason, they should be kind and strong enough to guide the patient if needed.

Futility

Treatment decisions can be difficult. When a clinician knows that active treatment is likely to be futile, it is only fair that she states this clearly. This can be extremely difficult for patients to hear and believe. Remember that public expectations are high, so the fact that nothing helpful can be done to cure the illness or to extend the patient's life is often very shocking information. When clinicians have to make this decision, it is also very difficult for them. All doctors want to help in any way they can, and when they are faced with telling a patient and his carers that there isn't a helpful treatment, their agenda has moved from organising treatment to breaking bad news. This is discussed in more detail later.

The important point here is that there is always something that can be done to palliate, relieve symptoms, and support the patient and his carers. The fact that treatment won't help will require careful explanation; it may also need examples, simple statistics, and a description of the burden of possible/likely side effects. Few people would want to spend a shortened life feeling so ill that they were unable to enjoy any aspect of living, especially if this is within the confines of a hospital environment, struggling with the symptoms caused by the toxic side effects of futile treatments.

When this is carefully and clearly explained to patients, they often agree with an agenda of best supportive care. However, as a species human beings are not designed to give up. It is unthinkable and sometimes even when faced with clear information of likely very poor response rates, a patient and/or his carers will insist on trying the treatment, even if the research shows a response rate of only 10%. It is fair to state that a clinician may see the response rate as a 90% chance of increased illness and likely earlier death and that the patient and his carers may see only a 10% chance of extended life. The tensions of opposing thoughts are extremely difficult for any clinician to handle. Often the main guiding ethical principle for doctors is 'Do no harm'. Doctors do not have to prescribe any treatment or intervene in any way that they consider to be futile. Whilst patients have the legal right to refuse treatment, they do not have the right to demand treatment. Their family has the right to either refuse or demand treatment (the exception is that of a lasting power of attorney, who may refuse a particular prescription for a patient who lacks capacity).

Treatment decisions belong to the doctor, by law. That they are discussed clearly and sensitively with the patient and his carers is good practice, requiring immense skill.

JONATHAN'S STORY

Bernice had inoperable cancer of the pancreas, which had spread to her liver. She was 60 years old, frail, jaundiced, and already symptomatic from liver disease. Her recent blood tests were bad, showing that her liver was failing. I had already met Bernice and her two supportive sons, and I was aware that they were hoping for a solution, for treatment.

There wasn't any that would be helpful. As Bernice and her family entered the consultation room, it was clear that she had become frailer; her mobility was reduced, and she had clearly lost weight. Whilst this made my decision easier, it didn't make the consultation easier. I know from experience that patients and particularly their carers don't see what we see as clinicians. I understand and respect that.

I invited them in and shook hands with Bernice and both her sons. 'Please take a seat', I offered warmly. 'Bernice, how are you feeling?' I asked.

'I just feel so weak, Doctor, and I feel sick all the time', she answered.

Her son Keith spoke immediately. 'Don't worry, Mum, that's why we are here, so the doctor can sort it out'.

Tony, his brother, joined the conversation: 'Remember Bob at our place, Mum? I told you about him; he had cancer, and he is doing great now, had the all clear'.

As predicted, I was faced with two loving sons, both expecting a solution and harbouring unrealistic expectations because of their experiences with a different cancer and limited knowledge. I expected it and completely understood it. No one is cancer wise until after the event. Being a cancer expert is my job and my responsibility. I maintained eye contact with Bernice and said, 'Bernice, it doesn't surprise me that you feel so poorly, I have the results from your last blood tests and they show that your liver is not working properly, which is why you feel so ill. I am sorry, but this is a worrying sign. I am afraid that the cancer I talked about in your pancreas is growing'.

Tony was undeterred, although I could tell from his facial expression that the word *worrying* had registered. He immediately asked, 'When can you start treatment, then, Doctor?'

I have learnt that a pause, just a moment's silence, is useful; it acts as a warning shot for the patient and her carers, and it allows me time to frame my reply. 'I am so sorry, Bernice, but chemotherapy is unlikely to help; the response rates are poor; only 10% have their life extended, by just a few months at best. The treatment would make you very ill, and I just don't think you are strong enough for it. Your liver wouldn't cope, and we would risk damaging your quality of life or, worse, shortening your life further'.

I sat quietly to allow my words to be absorbed. Bernice didn't seem surprised. I often think that because the patient is the one feeling so ill, and they realise just how ill they actually are, the thought of feeling even worse is unthinkable. Keith and Tony felt differently; it was obvious that they saw not having treatment as giving up, and they couldn't bear that thought. It was easy to see that their acceptance of my advice would seem as though they were giving up on their mum. 'Come on, Mum, you have to try, if 10% do okay, you will be one of the 10%, you just need to eat more, build yourself up, and keep fighting Mum', Tony pleaded.

I allowed Bernice to answer: 'I don't want it, Tony. I don't want to feel worse and end up in hospital, just for the sake of a few months. I just want to enjoy what bit of life is left now. He didn't talk of cure, you know'.

Keith supported Tony's view: 'Come on, Mum, you can't give up'.

It went quiet, as the three of them thought the unthinkable. I sat quietly with them, watching their faces and the changes in their expressions and the revealing looks between them.

I chose my next words carefully. 'Bernice, I think your agreement with this decision is both brave and right for you. Although we can't offer any treatment to extend your life, there is so much we can do to improve the quality of your life'. Tony and Keith looked so defeated and frustrated; it was right that I speak to them directly. 'Tony, Keith, I can see how hard this is for you, I'm so sorry that I can't help more. But it is my job to give you the best advice, and if it helps, if this was my mum, I would have chosen not to have the treatment for her'.

As always, this struck a chord; their eyes jumped from their laps to my eyes.

'Really?' they asked.

'Yes', I confirmed. 'It is important that your mum enjoys her life as much as possible and has a good quality of life with her family at home. There are so many people to help her with that. We will ensure that she is as comfortable as possible, for as long as possible. Our aim is still to keep mum here for as long as possible. Whilst we can't cure, we will support and treat all symptoms'.

Whilst the three of them looked defeated, the reality of the situation was sinking in. I could see them adjusting their expectations, and gentle supportive looks passed between them.

The decision was made, I had done my part of the job, and I showed them into a room to chat with the palliative care specialist nurse who would outline the support available. All three of them shook my hand and said, 'Thank you'. That always feels strange to me, being thanked for giving devastating news, but I have learnt that, horrendously difficult as it can be, if I have done my best, been clear, kind and honest, I can't do more than that. For Bernice, this was the right decision; there were 25 other patients waiting in my clinic, and they would all be different.

Jonathan's story shows how difficult it can be to inform a patient and his carers that treatment would be futile. People have such high hopes and are not designed to give up. Instinctively, they will try anything. It shows that it is helpful for the doctor to make the decision, not the patient. It would be too much of a burden to expect the patient and his carers to make a clinical decision when they do not have the scientific knowledge to make it; in fact, it would be cruel. The fact that Jonathan empathised with them, by mentioning how he would feel if it was his own mother, clearly helped Bernice and her sons. Patients and their carers can forget that professionals are also part of families and that they may have had similar experiences. They often assume that such things haven't happened to them, and for the professional to mention how they might feel if it were their relative can help enormously. It shows understanding and respect for how hard the decision is and supports the carers as they support the patient.

Jonathan used silence really well to allow information to sink in. His responses were well thought out, clear, and to the point. Ambiguous terms don't help; they serve only to distract from the decision-making process by offering a temporary escape route, therefore making it harder for everyone concerned. Crucially, Jonathan stressed what can be done rather than what couldn't be done and facilitated the appropriate support systems. At that point, as Jonathan said, his job was done and he moved on, to focus his attention on the next patient.

Clinical Responsibility and Support

All professionals are aware of the huge responsibilities they carry. Jonathan's story highlights this nicely. At the point of diagnosis and treatment planning, patients are feeling a huge array of emotions, including, for example, acceptance, adjustment, fear, anxiety, and hope. They feel lost in a system that is usually alien to them. No one wants to be a patient and they find themselves having to learn things they wish that they had never had to know about.

Hospitals are the comfort zone of professionals; patients usually have little understanding of how they function. It is vital that professionals understand this and explain the healthcare systems and professional roles to the patient at the time of diagnosis and, crucially, at the start of treatment.

For Bernice, as illustrated, this has fallen to the palliative care nurse specialist. Her task will be to introduce herself and allow time for Bernice and her sons to adjust to the information given in their consultation with Jonathan. There will be questions forming in their minds, and it is so important for them to have this time to frame their questions and decide on what they want/need to know at this time.

Allowing them to ask these questions is a good way to start a supportive interview. It provides an opportunity for the professional to show empathy and demonstrate good listening skills and knowledge from the outset. The patient and his carers can set the agenda and their priorities. Whether the patient is to start active treatment, e.g., chemotherapy or radiotherapy or a programme of best supportive care, the objectives will be the same for any professional involved. Often this will be to ask for an explanation of what the patient has just been told. Crucially, it gives the professional a chance to concentrate the agenda on what can and will be done to support the patient.

It is vital that the nurse works with the same agenda as the consultant who has just seen the patient. A dialogue that is congruent with the last conversation serves to make the patient and his carers feel safer within the system. The nurse can pick up on the patient's concerns and answer in a way that demonstrates that, as professionals, we share the same goals for patient care.

Answering the questions chosen by the patient and his carers ensures that they have understood what has just been said to them. Explaining what the consultation meant for them is vital. They need to know what will happen next and 'who' is responsible for 'what'. The following case studies demonstrate the skills needed.

GILLIAN'S STORY

It was obvious that Bernice, Tony, and Keith had understood what Jonathan had said to them. Bernice had clearly taken the role of supporting her sons, who seemed understandably stunned. Following on from Jonathan, I introduced myself. 'My name is Gillian. I work with Jonathan. I am the palliative care nurse'. I offered good eye contact and a warm smile as I directed them to their seats. 'How are you feeling?' I asked them.

Tony answered first: 'We are just shocked that nothing can be done; there must be some treatment, chemotherapy or something?'

Bernice spoke immediately: 'Tony, that would make me worse probably, he explained that, and I don't want all that messing, just to get a few more months, even if it works. I'm okay, love. This way is better for me; we all have to go sometime, love'.

Tony and Keith were struggling to control their tears, tears that clearly indicated that they were adjusting to reality. It always feels so much harder to see a man cry, even though in my job we see it all the time. Men are more solution-orientated than women and therefore find it so much harder to accept that there is no curative treatment available. The honesty and tears were a clear sign of the start of acceptance.

My role was to explain the key points of the consultation and to ensure that they felt supported. I started by using some of Jonathan's words. 'Jonathan mentioned to you that there is a lot that we can do, in terms of improving and maintaining your quality of life. Our aim is still to keep you here and feeling as well as possible, for as long as possible'.

Bernice smiled, and her sons waited for me to speak again. 'Your GP and community nurse are your key people; they have responsibility for your care at home. Your community nurse will come to visit and introduce themselves and will leave you with contact numbers should you need any help. They will also provide any hands-on care that is needed and organise any equipment to help you at home. Whilst they are not with you 24 hours a day, there will always be someone you can contact for help. My role as a specialist nurse is to support you with specialist problems related to your disease. There may be times when your medicines need adjusting to relieve symptoms, or you may need to chat things through and ask questions. Often, your GP and community nurse manage your care so well that I may not be needed, but there may be times when you or your community nurse feels that it will be helpful to see me. Jonathan will write to your GP, and I will speak to your community nurses; they will ring you to arrange when they can visit you'.

They nodded their understanding and I spoke again. 'I am so sorry that this has happened to you, but we will help you all we can'. I paused for them to absorb the information I had just given them. 'You mentioned to Jonathan that your main problems were feeling tired and constantly nauseated; could you tell me more about this, Bernice?'

Bernice was happy to talk about this: 'It takes me ages to get going in the morning, and I feel so sick. I manage bits of food, but feel sick afterwards and it gets worse as the day goes on'.

I answered reassuringly: 'Both those symptoms are common with this illness and there are medicines that I think will help with the nausea and we can arrange a prescription for those today. Tiredness is hard to cope with, there are no medicines for that sadly, but if we chat about how you can manage it and perhaps change your daily routine, it may help'.

Bernice was clearly happy to try any treatment to help with the nausea, and her sons sat quietly while Bernice and I chatted about how awful her fatigue was and how she could change her daily routine to better accommodate this. I could sense the weariness in all of them. I began to bring the meeting to a close. 'What would help you most today?' I asked.

'Getting rid of this nausea really', answered Bernice.

'Well, let's concentrate on getting you feeling better then', I offered in a positive tone. I organised and gave them a prescription for some anti-sickness medicine and gave them contact numbers for both the specialist nurse and the community nurse. 'Your community nurse will contact you and I will be in contact to ensure that your new medicines are helping. This has been a hard day for you and it is a lot to take on board. If you think of anything you want to ask me, please ring me, I will always return your call, and if I am out when you ring, you can leave a message. My working hours are on the card and leaflet I have given you'.

Bernice and her sons gathered themselves to leave; we shook hands and smiled at each other as they left. They thanked me, and I knew this was the start of a relationship where I would be needed, alongside their GP and community nurse.

HELEN'S STORY

I always feel it's so hard for patients at the start of their treatments, being thrust into this new world of clinics and so on. Tracey has breast cancer; she has had surgery and is about to start her chemotherapy, and she is scared. We had met at the time of her diagnosis. She spoke immediately: 'Hi, Helen, I am starting treatment next week;

I will feel better then, knowing that something is fighting the cancer. Is there any-thing I need to be doing?'

I chose a directive, clear approach to a clear question. 'Apart from looking after yourself well, no, lots of fruit and vegetables, decent food, and get lots of rest. Obey the messages your body gives you. This treatment is tiring; don't be afraid to give in and rest more. The chemotherapy team will contact you about your appointment for treatment and you will see the consultant regularly'.

'Will do', said Tracey, clearly wanting to help herself as much as possible.

'There will be lots of clinic appointments for blood tests, scans and treatments', I warned her.

'I don't mind that', answered Tracey.

I reassured her: 'We will be keeping a close eye on you and talking to you about your treatment regularly. You know how to contact us, don't you?' I asked.

'Yes, I have all the numbers', Tracey answered.

'They can be long days, Tracey, when you come to the clinic, and it gets harder, the more treatments that you have; don't be afraid to call for help', I told her.

'I won't'. She smiled as she got up to leave.

'See you soon and ring any time', I prompted as she left.

Whilst Bernice and Tracey were in different circumstances, both professionals involved used similar skills. Gillian concentrated on supporting the process of adjustment to no curative treatment and Helen outlined the process of active treatment whilst reassuring Tracey of the support that would be available to her throughout treatment.

The meeting between Bernice and Gillian began with Gillian continuing the agenda set by Jonathan and she concentrated on trying to fix what could be fixed, i.e., the nausea. This showed from the start that, as a professional, there is always something we can do to help and that Bernice would still be cared for. It helps dispel that awful feeling of leaving the consultation thinking that nothing can be done. Gillian showed that there is something that can be done to support the patient and her carers and ensure that they know that the professionals will work to improve and maintain the quality of life for the patient.

Gillian showed kindness with both her words and her use of silence; the patient and her sons set the agenda and were able to ask questions. When they left Gillian, they knew which professionals would be supporting them and had an outline of the different roles. This can be confusing information and crucially Gillian made sure she acknowledged this and encouraged them to contact her with any questions. Whilst it may seem harsh to ask directly, 'How are you feeling?' it does help patients to concentrate on considering their own emotions and questions, and they are grateful for this. It shows that the professional is interested in their thoughts and feelings and allows them to concentrate on what their main concerns are, and these concerns always vary. When Gillian focused on Bernice's symptoms, it showed that she had been listening and was aware of what was troubling Bernice. It also gave her an opportunity to demonstrate an important part of her role and begin a process of clinical management and support that Bernice and her sons would need from her. It may seem surprising for Gillian to say, 'I am sorry', but it is a human touch. Saying sorry is often associated with accepting responsibility, but when Gillian says, 'I am sorry that this has happened to you', it is a genuine, useful and kind acknowledgement of the harshness of the situation. Bernice and her sons left Gillian feeling understood, sup-ported, and clearer about who would be supporting them and how.

Helen quite rightly took a more directive approach. Whilst counselling is often patient/client-centred, there are times when the patient and his carers need clear direction from the professional as they try to understand their situation and the systems that are new to them. Helen, like Gillian, ensured that her patient understood what would happen next and crucially she warned Tracey of how hard it could be to be on a treatment regimen. Patients have usually not been in this position before and the many and various hospital appointments can be very taxing to their levels of energy and mood. It was important that Helen warned Tracey of this and gave her permission to rest and call when in need. For patients having active anticancer treatment, their response to this treatment has to be monitored, and they are often restaged with repeat scans. Helen warned Tracey of the ongoing management and tests that would be needed. There are often many outpatient appointments for the patient and her carers to endure. Whilst they do usually get used to it and usually appreciate it, it was so helpful that Helen talked openly and honestly about how hard it can be. Two very different situations where two different professionals offered relevant support by being clear, kind, and reassuring. Both patients left those meetings understanding their treatment plans and knowing which professionals would be involved and the differences in those professional roles. A contract was made with each patient about ongoing care, and both were assured of the professional's future availability.

It is so important that there are other professionals in supportive roles to work with the patients. It is a fact that doctors are often overworked and running very busy clinics, so time is often short. What isn't true, however, is that doctors don't want to ask about the patient's feelings and offer the necessary support. Often during the many follow-up appointments that patients attend, it is the patients who organise the consultation, to keep the doctor on the treatment agenda. They often want the doctor to see them as robust enough to continue treatment and do not want to distract the doctor by discussing their feelings. Instead, they will usually prefer to have these discussions with the professionals working alongside the doctors. During the active treatment stage, this approach works well. However, it may need to change in light of a poor response to treatment.

> TIP: *Waiting for feelings to be expressed may result in lost opportunities to express concerns – consider exploring pre-emptively.*

7

The Impact of Serious Illness

Uncertainty seems to be the hardest experience of all for the psyche to bear.

Change can be stressful. Negative change can be catastrophic. When patients are told that the treatment hasn't worked or that the situation is far worse than originally thought, the ground shifts beneath them and those who love them; everything changes; and that change can seem sudden to the patient and his family. Crucially, it is at the point of recognising the threat of serious illness that the patient's communication style may also change. An adjustment begins, which can be tangible to the professional listening, as she watches the patient absorb often devastating information.

ANNE'S STORY

I had been worried about Arthur; he had seemed unwell recently and had become increasingly breathless. Arthur was due to see the medical oncologist for a treatment review, and I made sure I was around to catch him after that consultation. I met him in the corridor waving his goodbyes to the staff; he greeted me warmly as Arthur always does. 'Hello there, Anne, good news! The cancer is progressing, and they have stopped the treatment. I just have to come back if my breathing gets worse. That's good news, isn't it?'

I had been expecting this. Arthur had had two cycles of chemotherapy and then a repeat chest X-ray, and the results of this had been explained to him today. It was, in fact, the opposite of good news, but given the ambiguity of words, it was understandable that Arthur had not understood what had been said to him at all. Radiological evidence of disease progression is bad news, the treatment had been stopped because it hadn't worked, and the cancer had grown during the treatment. There was no point in attending busy oncology clinics any more. The kind and supportive medical advice had been for Arthur to live his life but know that when his symptoms got worse (and they would), he could return to the clinic for the consideration of radiotherapy treatment and/or changes to his medicines to help relieve those symptoms. That was the sad reality, and it didn't match the look of cheer on my patient's face at all. It wasn't that Arthur was being unrealistic (which can sometimes be the case), he had genuinely not understood what had been said to him. I knew Arthur well enough to know his preferences in communication. Much earlier in our patient-to-professional relationship, he had told me clearly that he was a man who liked to know the truth and that he was philosophical about dying.

DOI: 10.1201/9781003427377-7

I guided him into an empty consultation room for a chat and told him clearly that when the cancer progresses, that isn't good news. I paused while he considered and continued by saying that *progression* means growth.

'Of course, it does', he said as the explanation registered. 'And they have stopped the treatment because it wasn't working?'

I nodded and held his hand as he shook his head slowly. 'So, what happens now, Anne?' he asked. Arthur was so easy to talk to; this conversation would have been so much harder to have with someone with a different personality and attitude.

'It's time to rest, Arthur', I told him. 'To enjoy not having to endure the treatment. You will feel better without it, it was doing you more harm than good, and there is no point having toxic treatment in your body if it isn't working. The doctor is right about that, and if your breathing gets harder, there is so much we can do to help you. You have a good team around you, and we will be keeping our eye on you, and you know we will help you when you need it'.

'I know that, Anne; everyone has been marvellous'. Arthur smiled. 'I was warned this cancer was a tricky one right in the beginning, I knew that they couldn't cure it. It will be good not to feel ill with the chemo; it did knock me sideways. So then, onwards and upwards as they say; it's a good job you caught me, you know. I would have been telling my family the wrong tale altogether! Not to worry, pet, thanks for being there, again', he concluded.

'Arthur, ring me any time and please tell your family the same', I told him. 'If they want to ring me to ask anything, they can. I will ring you in a couple of days anyway, bye for now'.

Arthur shouted his goodbyes to the clinic staff and left as I tapped on the door of the consultant who had spoken to him. As a professional, I know how hard we try to get it right and how much the consultant in the clinic cares about the standards of his care and communication. I retold the whole story of what had happened with Arthur. We all learnt a lot that day, and every time we learn, we improve our practice, and that has to be a good thing.

Anne's story could have happened anywhere. All professionals use their own specific language. It becomes a comfort zone. The importance of context is made clear here. Progression is about growth when it is applied to cancer; the fact that it is progressing is a bad thing, yet how understandable that Arthur had taken the wrong message completely from such clear language. Arthur had even seen the fact that the treatment had been stopped as a positive thing.

Anne's approach was tailored to Arthur's needs, a patient she knew well. Her style was kind, clear, and confident. She was able to explain the consultation without putting the doctor in a negative light as this would not have helped Arthur at all. A misunderstanding had occurred, which taught everyone involved a valuable lesson. It wouldn't be fair to conclude that the communication was a mistake, but it could have been done better. That is something that the consultant involved will have immediately thought when Anne retold the story to him. His tone and body language may not have matched the meaning of the words; maybe he didn't pause to evaluate whether his patient understood what had been said. Anne took a non-judgmental approach to her colleague. As far as he was concerned, Arthur had understood accurately and so had no questions to ask. Therefore, the consultant would not have seen the need to explain his X-ray results differently.

The most important thing Anne did was to focus on the positive, on what could and would be done. When treatment is stopped or a prognosis changes for the worse, patients can feel abandoned. Often, they have been attending clinics for treatments and consultations regularly and sometimes for a long time. It is understandable that they have learnt to rely on these hospital attendances and on the relationships that they have built with the staff there. To be told that they no longer have to attend hospital clinics can be both baffling and scary. What makes perfect sense to a clinician can confound a patient. Anne reassured Arthur clearly of ongoing support for both him and his family. She pointed out the physical benefits of not having to endure toxic treatments. There are real benefits: the body will have a chance to rest and recover, and Arthur can lead his life without incorporating hospital appointments into his routine. Due to their long relationship, Anne could judge how to communicate with Arthur, and Arthur was certainly easy to talk to.

As everyone is different, it is important to consider some of the other normal reactions that may occur when patients are told that treatment has stopped. It is not unusual for patients to feel very let down by the system when appointments and/or treatment are stopped. Seeing a doctor can be very reassuring for patients and crucial to their well-being. Questions such as 'How will I know what is happening to the cancer if there are no more scans and appointments?' are common. Or even, 'So I am just left to it now, am I?' Patients and their families can be apprehensive and this is exacerbated when hospital visits are reduced.

They can be fearful to the point of seeming angry, and it's vital that professionals recognise this and discuss the impact of these decisions at the time and offer a clear rationale for the decision.

It is very difficult for patients and their families to understand that clinicians will not order scans when there are no further treatment options. Such expensive investigations are used for diagnostic and treatment planning reasons. Of course, if the patient presents with fresh symptoms, which may indicate a new problem that can be treated, such as back pain suggesting malignant cord compression or the development of ascites which may be amenable to drainage (to give just two examples), there may be more investigations, but the routine tests to monitor the response to treatment which has now stopped are no longer needed and, crucially, would no longer be helpful.

It can take time and a gentle explanation for the patient and his family to accept this decision. Often, it is a difficult conversation, which may leave the patient feeling very upset. However, being emotionally upset is a clear sign that he has heard the information, and it has been understood. It takes time to adjust to negative information and expressions of emotion are often the start of that adjustment. It is very difficult for patients to imagine that professionals will still support them even when they don't attend clinics. The networks and professionals may be completely new or already known to them but will change shape around them to support new circumstances.

It is not unusual for specialist palliative care professionals to be introduced at such times. The patient may have had a long relationship with a particular professional, such as the breast care nurse, and it may be that the expertise of another professional such as a specialist in palliative care is now needed. Introducing a new professional to a patient requires skill. The explanation given has to be clear and the fact that it is in the patient's best interests understood. The knowledge base of each specialist is deep, due to the fact that they have concentrated their practice and applied their studies in one area. The patient can (when carefully encouraged to) apply this concept to other areas of his life, but there is no emotional attachment to the mechanic or plumber, and a change in professionals can, at first, be just another loss to them.

The introduction and assessment skills outlined in previous chapters are crucial. If a professional builds a therapeutic relationship at a time of need, the patient and his family soon adjust to the new relationship and appreciate the value in it. Initially, they cannot imagine what the professional knows by experience. It takes time, kindness, and guidance for the patient and his family to settle with and feel safe with a new professional. A pivotal issue is the timely transfer of relevant clinical information between professionals. Quite often, the professionals will work alongside each other.

Their different roles and knowledge bases may be needed and often the patient himself will make the transition from making one professional the first point of contact instead of the other in his own time. It doesn't matter whom the patient chooses to ring first if the professionals are liaising effectively to share care for the patient. Mutual respect, common sense, and effective communication prevent most problems from occurring in such circumstances. No professional should feel ownership over a patient; parochialism is divisive to patient care.

However, services for patients with non-malignant disease also include clinical nurse specialists. It is so important to consider the particular difficulties often presented to professionals who care for this group of patients, for example, those with chronic obstructive pulmonary disease (COPD) and heart failure. COPD is an umbrella term for a group of lung diseases that include chronic bronchitis, emphysema and small-airways disease. Lung damage over a long time impairs the flow of air in and out of the lungs and causes breathlessness. COPD is the fifth-biggest killer in the UK and the fifth-biggest killer worldwide.[1] Every hour, COPD is estimated to kill over 250 people worldwide.[2] Heart failure accounts for at least 5% of medical hospital admissions in the UK and up to 16% of patients are back in hospital within 6 months of their first admission. Prognosis is poor, on the whole, with 5-year mortality rates varying from 26% to 75%.[3]

When patients present with acute pulmonary oedema their prognosis is poorer; survival rates are predicted by severity. In those presenting with cardiogenic shock (hypotension with systolic blood pressure <90 mmHg, oliguria, and low cardiac output), hospital mortality can be as high as 90%.

The term *heart failure* is so absolute that alternatives such as *impairment* or *damage* may be preferred, but the risk is that some patients may feel patronised, and it is also reminiscent of times when the word *cancer* was avoided whilst talking to patients. Explaining that the heart is not pumping as strongly as it should is understood by nearly all patients and is a good starting point from which to elaborate and give further information as required. As ever, know your patient and communicate accordingly. A poor prognosis is inevitably attached to non-curable diseases, which therefore lend themselves well to clear, helpful discussions at the time of diagnosis. It is so helpful to all concerned and can prevent and reduce the stress of later discussions. Advance care planning is therefore discussed in detail later in the book.

Non-malignant diseases such as COPD and chronic heart disease have a different illness trajectory from cancer; for this group of patients, multiple admissions with frequent exacerbations necessitating complex treatment are the norm. This will inevitably have entailed numerous difficult discussions and decisions between the professionals, the patient and his family. It can therefore be much harder for the patient and his family (and even his doctors) to accept that the patient's condition has reached an end stage.

So much has been done to maintain his quality of life and so many admissions to hospital have improved the patient's condition that when such measures are no longer helpful, it can be too much for the patient and his family to accept.

It may be kinder to discuss end-of-life care under the umbrella term of *advanced disease* in the first instance to allow the patient and his family to adjust to the necessary change in the focus of care. However, the focus of care must change, and clear and kind discussions will be the responsibility of all professionals involved. Such discussions will need to include discussions about strategies for future care. The next exacerbation of illness may need to be managed differently to maximise the patient's quality of life. The clinicians, and indeed the patient, may feel that repeated admissions to hospital are no longer in the patient's best interests. Community professionals and specialists can provide care in the home, in order that hospital admission, where the patient would be at risk of hospital-acquired infections or may die in a place not of his choice, can be avoided. The focus of communication should always be on living life to the full for as long as possible, but openness about the reality of the situation, and the patient's condition, is crucial. As diseases progress and exacerbations increase for those with chronic illness, the sad reality is that patients are more likely to die. Honest conversations enable patients to express their own wishes and priorities and for their families to adjust or amend their behaviour and attitudes in light of this information.

BETTY'S STORY

After Ted died, the nurse said she hadn't wanted to tell me everything because she thought I would constantly worry about Ted gasping for breath, but I was worrying about this anyway, all the time. Not talking about it didn't stop me worrying at all. I lived with him 24 hours a day. I was the one sat with him, watching him sat on the edge of the bed trying to catch his breath. I tried really hard to encourage him, to keep his spirits up and not give in. If I had known he could die at any time, I would have been more patient with him, not pushed him to try as much. As it is, I look back now and wish every day that I had been kinder to him.

Betty's story illustrates well the valuable work that can be done by professionals when discussing the impact of serious illness. Professionals have a responsibility to share information with the patients and those who care for them, be clear and honest in their dialogue, and remember that, as professionals with a wealth of experience, it is likely that they have insight and knowledge that the patient and his carers don't have but would benefit from. Professionals are also aware of the stresses that can be part of the bereavement phase.

Guilt can be avoided or minimised by guiding families to alter their perspective at the right time, and this honesty can impact hugely on how people grieve.

No one should feel that they weren't informed of how bad the situation was. Gentle guidance and information giving are core components of every professional's role. Offering knowledge that may be 'new' to the patient allows him to alter future expectations and to accept new professionals being involved and a change in the care provided. 'When your problems change, your treatment and care will change alongside' – this reassuring sentence prepares the patient and his family for the dynamic nature of illness and helps them to expect and understand the frequent changes to the patient's medicine regime and nursing care. Whilst a professional will know how symptoms continually change and how the drug regimen must therefore be altered to relieve symptoms, the patient and his family do not and will require explanation and clarification.

Dementia

Dementia is a growing challenge as people live longer. It has become one of the greatest health and social care issues faced by the world. More than 55 million people have dementia worldwide. Every year there are 10 million new cases.[4]

There are currently 900,000 people living with dementia in the UK, and this is projected to rise to 1.6 million by 2040. The scale and the need to prevent, diagnose, support, live, and die well with dementia will only become greater.[5]

In summary, dementia is an overarching term that refers to a range of symptoms affecting cognitive abilities, while Alzheimer's disease is a specific type of dementia characterised by progressive memory loss and cognitive decline. Other types of dementia exist, each with its own distinct causes and characteristics.

DENISE'S STORY

Dad had died 6 months earlier. Mum had been getting worse from both understanding and memory points of view. It was getting harder, much harder.

Every night she woke me up to ask where Tom was; strangely, she never said, 'Where's your dad'. It was always Tom. Mum and Dad had been married for 70 years, and now she was totally lost.

It felt cruel to lie and cruel to keep repeating the bad news on a daily basis. It felt pitiful, painful, and impossible to protect her from anguish. Mum's anguish was worse when she realised that she didn't know. The worst anguish was because she couldn't remember and she would wail, 'Why don't I know this, where was I?'

I would tuck her up in bed with me and talk her through Dad's death, how she was with him all the time, how she told him she loved him and held his hand, and, most of all, how peacefully he died with her in his arms. This would settle her. She needed to know that she had done the right thing and that she had been with him. Cognitively, she still had the ability to understand that he was old and that his death was expected. Being reminded that **she had** been there was the most important thing, and she would settle.

Sadly, this scenario repeated regularly, she struggled to recognise the world without him in it. I would regularly talk to her about Dad, play the recording of his voice and reminisce until we laughed; this definitely helped. To keep him close comforted her, it kept her with him. Every night, she would say goodnight to his photo. People die; love does not.

Every patient with dementia will have their own unique difficulties; those closest to the patient, the carer, will have the best insight into their problems and will have *learnt strategies to mitigate them.*

Caring for someone with dementia is absolutely exhausting mentally, physically, and emotionally, and support services and social care are under-resourced.

It is vital that professionals learn from those who are the most involved with the patient's care, this may be the family at home or the staff in care homes.

The advent of Dementia UK and The Alzheimer's Society and their specialist nurses have made a huge difference. Both charities offer excellent resources to guide professionals through the stages of managing dementia.

It is important never to ask direct questions to people with dementia, to never ask if they remember something; this is often beyond their cognitive capabilities. Try to work with what they do understand if possible. Never correct what they have said; this will only increase confusion and make them feel more isolated. Work within their level of capability when possible.

Communication with someone suffering with dementia requires the professional to be totally focused on the patient; calmness and smiling can help, and touching their arm if they are comfortable with this. Avoid distractions and use only short simple sentences allowing time for them to formulate a reply.

Consultations will, of course, take longer, many of these patients will also have other health problems and challenges such as cancer. Communicating with the person who has lasting power of attorney is, of course, mandatory.

As the seriousness of illness impacts the patient and his family, many aspects of their lives may change. Working roles/hours may need to be adjusted and the patient and/or his family may be entitled to more financial aid as the patient's condition deteriorates. The professionals involved can help with benefit applications or direct them to professional services that can advise on these very important issues. Thinking about financial considerations at a time of failing health may seem vulgar, but the contribution which a regular income makes to family life is crucial. Money worries can be a massive burden, and relieving as much stress as possible is part of the professional's role and facilitating financial help is always greatly appreciated.

Having honest discussions about the changes in the roles of the patient and his carers is often a difficult task. It is also a task that can be one of the most rewarding: to see patients and their families adjust their thinking and behaviour in a way that contributes to increased well-being and reduced stress levels. Redefining oneself, one's life and future requires immense personal fortitude. The adjustment is stressful and made so much easier by open and clear discussion.

GAIL'S STORY

I had a real soft spot for Jo, having been her specialist nurse for two years, since diagnosis. She was back in hospital; the secondary disease from her bowel cancer was now causing problems that needed a hospital admission to sort. She was always brave and cheery; she knew the ward staff well and did her best to accept her hospital ward as home, for a while. Jo was only 43 years old; as a single parent, she was very close to her teenage sons. Her most recent relationship had not been what she had hoped for, but because Jo was Jo, she still had hope for lots of things. Jo had a colostomy bag and catheter to endure and now she had been told that it was necessary for her to have a nephrostomy tube inserted to drain a non-functioning kidney.

I went into Jo's room, pulled up a chair, held her hand, and waited for her to choose what we talked about. She fixed her eyes on mine and said, 'Gail, I'll never have sex again', and she cried, a lot, as we sat in silence; she cried for the loss of her sexuality. She was so beautiful, had always been a live wire, a gorgeous-looking girl, and like all human beings, she needed to be touched and feel worthy, sexually desirable, and most of all loved. Her statement wasn't one I could challenge. In the absence of a caring and well-established relationship, I was sure that she was right, she probably would never have sex again. Acknowledging the pain of that realisation and allowing Jo to verbalise her feelings were the most helpful things I could do. I felt humbled that she had chosen me to cry with and recognised how hard it would have been to have had that conversation with her family. She knew that they would have perhaps considered that to be the least of her worries, as she embarked on yet further chemotherapy and dealt with the insertion of the nephrostomy tube, but to Jo, that day, it was huge. It was all she wanted to talk about and the reason that she cried all day. I remember saying, 'It's okay to cry, Jo, because that is worth crying for'. I tried to imagine how I would feel and guessed that I would have felt the same way and would also have been unable to talk to my parents, brother, or teenage sons about it. It was such a huge issue, and Jo's words and tears that day taught me more than anything I have read. I never forget to consider the impact of serious illness on a person's sexuality now. Amidst the clinical decisions and practice, that human element is always 'on my radar', thanks to Jo.

Serious illness can change the way a patient looks and feels, both in emotional and physical terms. From diagnosis, the patient may have endured surgery, chemotherapy and/or radiotherapy. They may have lost body parts, hair, and self-esteem. Treatments can be physically costly; anxiety, depression, and fatigue are particularly common and difficult to manage. Although healthcare professionals are now more aware of sexual concerns, many people continue to receive little or no information about sexuality during their treatment or illness. They may, in fact, have had no real opportunity to ask important questions. If sexuality has not been discussed with them or if their questions have been avoided, they may feel that their worries and questions are foolish, unimportant or perhaps inappropriate. It is so important that those feelings don't prevent the patient from seeking answers and helpful treatments or from being able to grieve for such an important loss. Signposting a patient to relevant professionals such as gynaecologists, sexual counsellors, and urologists, for example, or advising on appropriate treatments is invaluable. It may be, for example, that drugs are appropriate for some men suffering erectile dysfunction, and medical staff are always willing to consider this as an option unless medically contraindicated.

Patients are often keen to keep the doctor on the treatment agenda and may not mention this as a concern during their consultations. It is often supporting clinical staff (nurses or allied healthcare professionals) who pick up on this as a problem that is causing a lot of upset to the patient or are asked directly for help by them. For some patients, their sexuality won't be an issue or consideration, but if and when it is, professionals need to be sensitive and astute in their assessments and communication.

As a disease progresses, the problems it produces and the solutions to these problems change. Within the context of palliative care, inevitably, the time will come when patients and their carers have to face the challenges of dealing with a short prognosis.

TIP: When describing the progression of disease, always describe the positive influence of medication and supportive care. 'I'm not going to get better from this, am I?' – 'No, but we will always do what we can to keep you well, for as long as possible'.

References

1. National Statistics. *Health Statistics Quarterly 30*. Available at: www.statistics.gov.uk/downloads/ theme_health/HSQ30.pdf
2. World Health Organization. *The World Health Report 2002. Reducing risks, promoting healthy life*. Geneva: World Health Organization, 2002.
3. Cowie MR, Mosterd A, Wood DA, et al. The epidemiology of heart failure. *Eur Heart J*. 1997; 18(2): 208–225.
4. World Health Organisation, *Key facts dementia*, Geneva: World Health Organization, 2023.
5. Alzheimer's Society. *Local statistics*, London: Alzheimer's Society, 2024.

8

Confirmation of a Poor Prognosis

Accepting the unacceptable. … How do you stop searching for a solution?

Human beings are not designed to give up, not on themselves, not on those whom they love. There is no such thing as a disease of the spirit. Hearing that treatment is either not possible or has not been effective is horrendous news. Often this dreadful news is given after the patient has endured multiple treatments and coped with the side effects, in the fervent hope that he will be one of the successful statistics described by his clinician before treatment started. Alternatively, he discovers at diagnosis that there is no disease-modifying treatment and that time is short. This chapter discusses the conversations needed for the patient and his family when the unthinkable happens.

PETER'S STORY

I'd gotten used to consultations. It's amazing what you get used to! I used to sweat over every damn blood test and scan result, but as I got on with it, I got used to it. Either the surgeon or my oncologist always seemed to have something else up their sleeve, so I didn't mind. 'More chemo' – Yeah okay. 'I'm gonna just cut a bit of your liver away' – Fine, go ahead; you had a bit of my lung, go for it! So, they did, they got on with it, and so did I. For three years, through all the ups and downs, I managed, always rallied. You have to just keep carrying on.

Deep down, I knew it was bad from the start; mind you, they told me and believe me, I heard them, loud and clear at the time. Yet, as I went through the treatments, coped okay, and got good results, well generally, I started to feel a bit invincible, I think. There was always another option and I got used to it. I ignored the little voice at the back of my head; it didn't help to listen to it. Even now I think that. You have to be brave and positive to deal with this and just surrender your body to the experts. Now the experts tell me, 'That's it, Peter, no more treatment options; we can try and put you in a clinical trial, but the results are not good and we are worried it will do more harm than good'. Now, if my oncologist isn't hopeful, I am certainly not! No point is there? I just hope I haven't used up all my fighting spirit though; I still want to be around for as long as possible. I have a daughter to walk up the aisle; I daren't ask whether that goal is realistic today. I just need to take this in. I can't bear the thought of them looking after me. As sick of the wedding talk as I am, I don't want to shatter their plans with this. I don't know when to tell Maisie, she's due to get the all-clear for her breast cancer. It's a bugger when husband and wife share the same oncologist. This is the big one, eh, the-nothing-more-we-can-do? I can't imagine it. I look fine, just had a holiday, all tanned. 'You look well, Peter'. Yeah, right! This is the talk I dreaded, and all I feel is how, and when, do I tell my family? I just feel weird, it's a hell of a lot to take in.

DOI: 10.1201/9781003427377-8

Peter's story illustrates well many of the emotions and thoughts experienced when a patient has been told that time is now short, that he will die from this disease and soon. It can be too much to take in, and sometimes it can be confirmation of news that he has been preparing himself to hear. It is often easier for the patient to make sense of it when he is very symptomatic, but that is not always the case. Peter was feeling quite well; in his mind, his symptoms did not match the test results.

Conversations of this nature are as stressful as conversations relating to initial diagnosis. Peter's illness journey had been years long; he had become used to the next treatment strategy. Although he admitted that somewhere in the back of his mind he had expected and feared this eventuality, there is never, ever a good or right time to face it. No one wants to die, to not be here. Peter's first reaction was one of guilt, not wanting to spoil the wedding planning phase and desperately wanting, and needing, to be able to walk his daughter down the aisle. There will always be an event in the family that a patient is hoping to be alive for. Many people define themselves by the relationships they have and their role within those relationships. It is reasonable to want to protect those you love from the devastating news of a poor prognosis. The clinician had obviously given Peter clear information, he was reacting to it and considering what he wanted to do and say next.

It is sensible to allow time for this information to 'sink in'. Professionals will be available to talk again when Peter has internalised his thoughts and feelings. Hope does have to be just about fighting the disease. It can apply equally well to hoping for quality of life, to being well for as long as possible. Setting achievable goals is helpful, promising or implying that a patient can reach an unachievable goal isn't. Honesty and clarity from the communicating professional can alleviate any problems which may occur regarding this. Hopelessness is so difficult for human beings to bear. There must always be something to hope for. Encouraging patients to alter their hopes in the light of new information is an invaluable skill. It is helpful to think of an appropriate professional response to Peter's account.

POST-CONSULTATION SUPPORT

I'm sorry, Peter – really sorry – that this has happened to you. This is awful news, and I think you are right to take some time to absorb what has been said; there is no rush to discuss this with anyone. Take your time. It will be easier to talk to your family when you have got used to the news yourself. It will be hard to think straight for a while. You have managed so well so far, and it is likely the next phase won't be any different in that way. We will be there to help you. There is so much we can do to keep you feeling as well as possible, for as long as possible, and we can talk more about that another day. Not having the treatment will make life easier in a way. You have time to rest, look after yourself, and plan for what is important to you. If you want me to help you talk to your family or answer any of their questions, I will. Although we can't cure this, because you are well at the moment, we are still hoping for some good times for you and your family. This has been a horrible day for you, Peter, so I won't keep you. Is there anything you would like to ask me? Is there anything I can help you with today?

The preceding dialogue illustrates some of the salient points of such an important discussion. Peter's feelings and coping strategies have been normalised and approved.

This can help patients enormously; there are no right or wrong ways to react or behave. It helps to support their choices. The word *sorry* can be ambiguous and often applied to the more trivial matters in life, and some patients may respond to a professional saying they are sorry by saying, 'It's not your fault'. Here, the professional made it clear that she was sorry that this had happened to Peter; that expression contains kindness and clarity that are befitting to the gravity of the situation.

The professional has focused on the positive and reminded Peter of how well he has coped and managed his illness so far. To state that it is likely that he will continue to do this will give Peter confidence. The opinion of a professional, whom the patient knows and trusts, matters enormously to patients.

Indeed, it matters far more than the professional often realises. Reminding patients that they already have a working template/script that can be strengthening to the spirit and can remotivate them during the hardest of times. Essentially the professional has taken the fact that Peter is feeling well now and used it to exert a positive influence on the clinical situation: he is symptom-free, and that is always a good sign!

A crucial part of the discussion was the reference to planning, particularly to planning around Peter's choices. The professional offering her availability, and screening for questions, to make sure that he didn't have any problems requiring immediate attention, concluded the discussion well.

Of course, every situation is different, and there are those patients who do not feel well, for whom the information outlining a poor prognosis merely confirms what they were thinking or prompts them to ask for more treatment, any treatment.

The range of reactions is wide. Some patients may feel so ill at this point that they readily accept the futility of further treatment. This applies equally to patients with both malignant and non-malignant diseases. They are in desperate times and can seem so overwhelmed that psychological support for the patient and his family may need to concentrate on how they feel emotionally and allow them to cry and grieve for their future. Being vigilant and recognising where there may be solutions to problems will always be good practice.

JILL'S STORY

I felt so sad for Tommy. He was clearly overwhelmed, both emotionally and physically. Throughout the treatment, he had struggled to cope.

He had been so unwell, and the burden of toxicities had taken a toll on his frail body. I was relieved that the consultant had had a clear discussion with him and that treatment had been stopped. His generation can be so accepting, so polite and undemanding; I could see that the consultant had been humbled by Tommy's gratitude as he left the consultation room. Tommy didn't want to be a burden. 'I can see how busy you are, love. I'm okay; I'll see you soon', he said. But Tommy wasn't okay; he was far from okay. He had gulped and hiccoughed all through the consultation, he looked weak, frail, and unsteady. Worse still, he looked defeated. I sat him down, and I could see the relief immediately. Tommy needed extra care now, and that was obvious. I held his hand until I got eye contact.

'Tommy, if it's okay with you I'm going to talk to your GP and community nurse. I really think it would help if they popped in to see you. I can see things are getting harder and that you need more help. Is anyone at home today?' I asked.

'No, love; I'll be fine', Tommy answered. 'I just need to get home and get settled. I'm not going to worry my daughter tonight about it, and I will see her tomorrow anyway. By all means, talk to my doctor, but he can't do anything, can he?'

'Yes he can, Tommy; there is so much we can do to help you now; you mustn't feel you have to struggle alone', I assured him. 'I am going to organise a prescription today, some tablets that will help with the sickly feeling and those hiccoughs too. I can see that you are not feeling well, Tommy, and we are here to help you. Do you mind waiting while I organise a prescription for you?'

Tommy sat back down. 'Thanks, love', he murmured.

Jill's assessment of the situation and the interventions she made would have helped Tommy enormously. Whilst he felt defeated and that he had no alternative but to accept feeling so ill, Jill encouraged him to accept help from key professionals. She had picked up on his symptoms and intervened to organise a prescription that would relieve them. This action would give Tommy confidence in the palliation of his symptoms and discourage him from just accepting new or worsening symptoms in the future. There will always be patients for whom professionals need to be extra-vigilant, who need guidance through the support systems, and encouragement to complain of troublesome symptoms. There are those who will make contact readily and those who need regular monitoring because they are unlikely to complain. Being able to assess different attitudes in patients is a vital skill for all professionals. Being able to tailor communication to each individual can make the difference between providing optimal care and missing an opportunity to help someone who needs it.

Conversely, there will always be patients who request treatment that isn't compatible with sound clinical judgement. The thought of not having any treatment is just too difficult to bear; indeed, these patients are often very keen to try anything, sometimes to the point of being willing to die from the toxicities of treatment rather than accept what they see as 'giving up'. Discussing the futility of treatment with patients who are facing a poor prognosis is a difficult challenge for professionals. Families often have strong feelings about these issues. They may lead with their emotions during discussions and find it difficult to accept that they have no legal rights with respect to the patient's treatment. The skills needed to manage this challenge will therefore be discussed in the next chapter.

BETTY'S STORY: NUTRITION

I had suspected that the treatment hadn't worked and that they would stop it, but I was determined that Sam wouldn't give in easily. I felt that sometimes he had given up; he refused meals all the time. How was he going to fight the cancer without food? I couldn't bear it. Giving him the best food was all I could do then. We had started to argue about it a lot; he would shout, I would cry, and the family would come around and try to persuade him to eat more. It became an awful situation. I wasn't going to surrender; why was he?

As it happened, one day in the middle of one of our arguments, our doctor arrived. I explained how frustrated Sam made me, and both Sam and I burst into tears. I was so embarrassed at first. I thought the doctor would think I was a mean, impatient person, but he didn't: he was lovely to us. He said he saw this all the time in families, and that really helped me. He stayed such a long time that day and he told me that all carers do this, concentrate on the food thing, because we feel that's all we can do to help, but he let me know, kindly, that it wasn't helping. I knew that Sam was more ill, of course I did, but I forgot to think about how that might feel, that he just didn't have an appetite anymore and really couldn't help it. Apparently, eating more than he wanted to wouldn't have helped the illness anyway. I could see how relieved Sam was that the doctor had said this, and I felt guilty then, to be honest. Poor lad, feeling so ill, and having to put up with me nagging on top of it all. Then Sam felt guilty and sobbed again. 'I'm sorry, Betty, you are trying so hard, love, but I feel sick at the mention of food these days'. What a pair we must have looked like! It helped though: it helped so much. Our doctor explained why Sam had no appetite and why big meals wouldn't help. We were so relieved by the time the doctor left that day. No more arguing for me and my Sam, and we didn't either. I let him eat what he wanted, when he wanted. I'm so glad now, without that doctor, that day, we would have got ourselves more wound up and spent his last weeks at each other's throats.

Betty's story outlines a very common problem. Eating is a human element, firmly entrenched in our social lives. As human beings, we see food as a means of survival. It is extremely difficult for families to accept that their loved one no longer wants to eat in the same way. Sadly, it is not unusual for carers to add extra food and supplements to their diet. Whether these are ordinary foods or foods as advised on internet sites and/or supplements, all can be anxiety-provoking for the patient.

Terminal diseases adversely affect a patient's normal metabolism. The body does not use food in the normal way and patients are no longer able to utilise the nutrients in the food. Therefore, too much food becomes a physical and psychological burden to them, it increases their sense of failure and guilt by constantly having to apologise and explain their symptoms and lack of appetite. Such tensions are regularly seen by professionals and should always be addressed, either at the time of discussion regarding appetite or pre-emptively.

The problem is so common that it is advisable for professionals to raise this issue in their discussions about the changing phase of illness and care.

The explanations and reassurance given by professionals can defuse and prevent tension and upset in an already emotionally charged environment. This may not be an easy task for the professional. Patients, and particularly their families, can be very tenacious about concentrating on nutrition. Many discussions and consultations are taken up with the patient or carer reading a list of what has been consumed in the last 24 hours. Focusing the patient and his family on the most important issues of quality of life is a real skill, and repetition and patience may be needed here. Clear challenges to the fear of the patient 'starving' or 'wasting away' may have to be made.

Laypeople, usually, do not have the biological knowledge of diseases to understand what is happening in the body during the final months and weeks of life. They see food as a comfort and a remedy: a way of fighting the illness. Importantly, meals and eating are highly 'loaded' with emotional attachment. Memories are often made up of family events and celebrations where food was the main focus. It is very important to clearly state to the family that a carer cannot be a curer in these circumstances and that many or most patients with terminal illness ultimately are unable to eat enough to avoid weight loss and maintain activity levels. In most circumstances, they genuinely won't have realised this. Patients often have their own feelings of guilt and shame relating to the changes in their appearance. Feelings of 'wasting away' are typical and are particularly difficult for men to cope with. Honest discussions can help with this. In the same way that investigations are not done when treatment is stopped, advising patients not to weigh themselves is very helpful. Monitoring a patient's weight is clinically useful during treatment. At the point of confirmation of a poor prognosis, there is no longer any benefit in him weighing himself. With kind and clear communication, firmly held beliefs and attitudes can be altered to benefit a situation that is changing for the worse.

Whatever the pathology, the realisation of a poor prognosis requires the key element of planning. There can be no excuse for a professional not addressing this issue when the clinical situation is clear.

The surprise question: Would you be surprised if the patient were to die in the next 12 months?

If professionals ask themselves this question and the answer is no, then it is a clear indicator that end-of-life care planning is needed. It is also a very useful question for professionals to ask of other professionals involved in the patient's care. For example, a nurse may ask this question of a doctor, in an effort to concentrate the doctor's thoughts on changing care and interventions to suit the current phase of the patient's illness.

It is incumbent on all professionals involved in a patient's care to ensure that important information follows the patient. Jill made this point well when she made it clear that she would be alerting Tommy's GP and community nurses to his changing needs. For patients who are at home, there are important practical considerations to enable the patient to stay at home, if this is his wish.

Patients in the end-of-life phase of their illness are very likely to experience troubling symptoms at some time. Often this can happen when the key professionals (whom the patient knows well) are off-duty, for example, on weekends and during the night. Clear information and care plans should therefore be shared at the appropriate time. Communicating the right things is important; saying them at the right time and to the right people is crucial.

Written information should be sent to the out-of-hours service providers to inform them of the diagnosis, past and current treatments, recent symptoms, medicines available in the patient's home, telephone numbers of professionals involved, and, most importantly, the patient's wishes regarding care at the end of life.

STEVE'S STORY

Carl was 49 years old, and he had an awful, huge, fungating anal tumour. Sadly, the surrounding tissues had not healed from the surgery or the radiotherapy treatment, which the clinicians had done in order to try and control his disease. The tumour was infected and bled regularly and sometimes copiously. His community nurses were brilliant and went to Carl twice a day to dress the tumour and wound. Alongside their care, his girlfriend, Maggie, coped well with his failing mobility and need for high-dose analgesics. Everyone involved knew Carl well; he often needed our help, he was very clear about what he did and didn't want, and he didn't want to go back in hospital. This made planning his care much easier but caused some anxiety for the nurses who were 'less used to' end-of-life care.

The clinical situation was that the bleeding from the tumour may increase, and there was a risk that the bleed would be huge, even a catastrophic fatal event. I noticed in the community nurse's notes that Sally (one of the community nurses) had written, 'In the event of large anal bleed ring 999' (emergency services). As a more knowledge-able and experienced professional, I knew that there was no helpful clinical interven-tion available should this happen. It wasn't possible to intervene either surgically or medically to stop the bleed (should it occur). The patient and his carers should be at the centre of every decision, so I sat down to talk to Carl and Maggie.

I began with a question, to help Carl focus on the issue. 'Carl, the bleeding is get-ting worse, isn't it?' I asked.

'Yes, I know', answered Carl without anxiety.

It was easy to discuss this openly with him. 'Carl, we can't be sure, but this bleed-ing may increase; we can't say when, but it may do. If it does, there isn't any proce-dure that could stop the bleeding. There would be no point in you going to hospital to see surgeons. They would decide only to give you the medicines that we can give you here at home. If you bled to the point where you became unconscious, we could look after you here, where you want to be. I am not particularly expecting that to happen, but I know how you feel about hospitals and staying at home, and I wanted to have an honest conversation with you about it'.

'Suits me', Carl answered quickly. 'I am not going anywhere'.

Maggie looked anxious. 'Do you mean he might bleed to death?' she asked.

It is important to be clear and calm in these situations, so I answered, 'It is possible, Maggie, though not necessarily probable. The blood vessels are clearly leaking, the tumour has definitely made them bleed, and it could get worse or stop on its own or stop and start. We will continue to keep our eye on it. If Carl bleeds a lot, his blood levels may be so low that we have to organise a short stay in the hospice for a blood transfusion; I can talk to the medical staff if that happens. Sometimes a transfusion can help people feel better. What I am discussing is if Carl has a big bleed, which we can't stop, we would keep him in bed and comfortable; it is a very peaceful process. Sirens and emergency rooms are not peaceful and wouldn't help at all', I explained.

'I wouldn't go', interjected Carl.

Maggie was thinking hard. 'So what do I do if it happens?' she asked.

'Ring the community nurses', I answered. 'We have all the medicines here that they may need and they will come right away and make Carl comfortable, here at home, with his family. It will be fine, Maggie, and it may not happen at all. But it's important that we talk about it, in case it does. I will speak to the GP and the community nurses to tell them of our decision, and it will be written clearly in the community nurses' notes'.

Carl was relieved by the decision and agreed with the actions, and Maggie was calm at the end of the conversation. I spoke to the doctor responsible for Carl's care. We had discussed and agreed on this conversation before I had gone to see Carl, and he was pleased to hear that it had gone well. It was very important for me to ring Sally, the nurse who had written 'ring 999' in the notes. I knew Sally; she was a good nurse who worked hard to maintain high standards of care. She was always keen to do 'the right thing', and fear of litigation is an ever-increasing problem for health-care professionals. When I explained the decision to her and the reason for it, she completely understood. She was clinically astute enough to see that there would be nothing anyone could do to stop the bleeding and that an emergency transfer would put Carl with unknown professionals in a clinically hectic setting. She was grateful for my input and admitted that she wouldn't have felt confident enough to make that decision or to have that conversation.

As professionals, we work in teams, and we work together. End-of-life care, including difficult communication about ethical issues, is my comfort zone. I would have been less than useless at handling those dressings on a daily basis. Sally, the doctor, and I have mutual respect. We talk often, and crucially, we listen to Carl.

Good end-of-life care may include deciding not to embark on futile treatments or not to take inappropriate actions, respecting the patient's views and clearly recording decisions made. For Carl, his decision to stay at home should he bleed heavily was compatible with the clinician's opinion on the futility of treatment. As it was clearly discussed, recorded and agreed, amongst all those involved, further documentation wasn't required in Carl's case. However, there may be occasions when more structured documentation is needed.

Advance Care Planning

End-of-life care is high on the agenda of many Western governments and there is much guidance for professionals. Advance care planning is just one part of those initiatives. The key word is *planning*. The crucial requirement is that professionals plan and communicate well with patients, their families and all professionals involved.

Advance care planning (ACP) is a process of discussion with the patient and his care providers, irrespective of their discipline. The difference between ACP and more general planning is that it often takes place in the context of anticipated deterioration in the patient's condition.[1] It therefore allows for the patient to express his wishes on the type of care he receives at the time of death. It facilitates discussion and can lead to the documentation of a patient's wishes before mental capacity or the ability to communicate his wishes to others is lost or altered. These wishes can then be used to guide the care provided for the patient.

With the patient's permission, those wishes should be documented, shared with the key professionals involved in the patient's care, and regularly reviewed. The patient's family or friends may be involved in these discussions at the request of the patient.

ACP discussions may include the patient's concerns, values and goals for care, his understanding of his illness and prognosis and the type of care and treatment that may be beneficial in the future and its availability. A statement of wishes and preferences may also be recorded. This is a broad term for a list that covers a patient's wishes, beliefs, and values and an explanation of how he has made the decisions which may govern future care. It is a record of written or verbal requests by the patient and may cover both medical and non-medical matters. It could be used when the patient has lost mental capacity. It is not legally binding but should be used to guide decisions that may be made for the patient in his best interests when he has lost the capacity to make those decisions.

Advance Decision

An advance decision must relate to a refusal of specific medical treatment and can specify circumstances. It will only come into effect when the individual has lost the capacity to consent to or refuse treatment. Careful assessment of the validity and applicability of an advance decision is essential before it is used in clinical practice. Valid advance decisions which are refusals of treatment are legally binding.

Lasting Power of Attorney

A lasting power of attorney is a statutory form of power of attorney created by the Mental Capacity Act.[2] Anyone who has the capacity to do so may choose a person (an 'attorney') to make decisions on his behalf if he subsequently loses capacity. The decision the person makes relates only to refusing treatment, not to demanding it.

In all cases, whatever style or form of communication is used, the following points may be worth considering:

- Do the patients and their families understand the clinical situation? Is further discussion needed?
- Do all the relevant professionals have clinically relevant and up-to-date information?
- Has the patient made a will, or does he need advice regarding his personal affairs?
- Do the patient and his family have realistic expectations and objectives?
- Are there any issues which the patient feels strongly about and therefore need to be formally recorded?

TIP: The more complex the situation, the more important it is to keep it simple.

References

1. NHS National End of Life Care Programme. *Capacity, care planning and advance care planning in life limiting illness: A guide for health and social care staff.* Available at: www.endoflifecareforadults. nhs.uk/publications/pubacpguide (accessed May 2011).
2. Department of Health. *The Mental Capacity Act.* Cm 11555. London: Department of Health; 2005.

9

Key Ethical Issues in Communication

Every situation within palliative care has the potential to present its own ethical dimensions and challenges.

The law and ethics are often discussed side by side, but they are very different subjects. The law will set clear boundaries relating to what a professional can and cannot do within her practice. Ethical principles will guide a professional to make judgements and decisions based on morals.

The key ethical principles as described by Beauchamp and Childress[1] are as follows:

- *Respect for autonomy.* This recognises the right of an individual to make decisions based on his own values. This requires a truthful exchange of accurate information about status, goals of care, options, and expectations.
- *Beneficence.* This is the most commonly used principle: to do good, namely, to do positive acts to maximise patient care.
- *Non-maleficence.* To do no harm, with either treatment or communication, and to consider the burdens and benefits for the patient of both.
- *Justice.* This may relate to fairness in the application of care, for example, the allocation of resources, including which patient gets a private room.

Many of these issues have already been touched upon as, unsurprisingly, they are woven within the routines of all healthcare work. This chapter discusses in more detail the difficult ethical problems that commonly arise in palliative care, and crucially, offers some guidance regarding helpful communication.

Autonomy

The translation *autonomy* from the ancient Greek is 'one who gives oneself their own law'.

In medicine, respect for the autonomy of patients is an important goal, although it can conflict with a competing ethical principle, namely beneficence.

 DOI: 10.1201/9781003427377-9

CAROL'S STORY

That day was one of my worst days, professionally, a day of constantly questioning myself and always reaching a self-damning conclusion.

As a clinical nurse specialist, I get to make decisions; sometimes those decisions, although discussed with others, can feel like lonely decisions. It's easy to talk to other professionals who you know are on your side; it's harder to answer the voices in your own head. When you care enormously about your patients and your practice, those voices are always there. The weight of the decision that I made that day reduced me to tears, tears that no one saw, as I led the decision and subsequent clinical care. That I make those decisions about clinical care and admissions is expected of me: it's my job that I sometimes agonise over. This is known and respected by some and unnoticed or unacknowledged by others. Such is the environment we all work in; it's understandable.

I had known Kim for 3 years, from when she had been diagnosed with breast cancer that had already spread to her chest wall and liver.

She was young, only 42 years old, and she had a young family: a 4-year-old boy. Due to the nature of her disease and the advances in treatment, I knew from the outset that it would be a long journey for us both. We always got on well, Kim and me. It can be hard to strike the balance of supporting during the bad times and retiring to the background when not needed. You often worry that the patient won't ring you when you are needed again; I never had that worry with Kim. She would always ring me, and it was always with good reason. If I rang her and all was well, she would hate to take up my time. We cried and laughed many times together and inevitably (as two mums) talked of many things. She had a childlike quality about her when she was scared, and she did get scared. She would raise her arms like a little girl to be hugged when I arrived, having taken a call from her and arranged a visit. Then we would sit, assess the problems, sort the medicines, run through the worries one by one, and always end with another hug. Kim hugged like a child, as though she was hanging on and soaking up some strength to use till next time. I didn't see her as a child, but those hugs often reminded me of when I had left my little girl at school, who didn't want to be there and would be waiting for me to go back and collect her.

Over the 3 years, Kim had shared many thoughts and feelings; I knew particularly that she wanted to be at home, with her husband and, crucially for her, with her little boy. We all worked hard to make that happen: she had a fabulous doctor and community nurses. Also, her oncologist in the hospital could not have been more helpful whenever I rang, and I did ring often: for scans or an appointment, for a review because recent clinical signs were worrying me.

I can see now that I started worrying before anyone else. I knew a year ago that things were starting 'to go wrong', because I knew Kim, and my frame of reference was more accurate, so when the scan results showed stable disease, I wasn't relieved. I could tell that soon the scans would match the change in symptoms that I could see. Sometimes it's an instinct thing – all experienced professionals have it. Kim's pain was complex, and her medicine regimen was equally so. It was a challenge and it got harder and harder to manage her symptoms, for all of us.

The consultants I work with were marvellous; they always are. Kim even agreed to come into the hospice more than once so we could try to improve things. Every time she couldn't get out quick enough, we all understood that. Every discharge had more concerns attached to it as Kim's symptoms escalated and her mobility and cognitive function deteriorated. A burden of diffuse disease can cause a huge burden of symptoms. It had become impossible to keep Kim biochemically stable, and any reduction in analgesics, which were causing sedation, resulted in an intolerable level of pain. Within this specialty, we accept that our patients will have complex needs, and we face the burdens-and-benefits debate of clinical decisions on a daily basis.

I had serious concerns about Kim's last discharge from the hospice, as did most of us. The whole team contributed to the decision and the organisation of services to support her at home. Kim was desperate to go home; she had mental capacity, and she had sound reasoning and was able to understand our concerns. Her conclusion after any discussion about our professional concerns relating to her discharge always resulted in the same answer from Kim: 'I just want to go home'. All the hospice-based professionals felt she should be discharged, as soon as possible. They felt it was her 'right', and it was our job to uphold that 'right'.

Although the community nurses and I had our worries, we agreed it was appropriate to support Kim to go home. I knew Kim's husband well. Chris was a devoted husband and dad, and he was scared, really scared about whether he would cope, but he wanted 'what was best for Kim'; he wanted to do whatever she wanted. Predischarge, we had lots of conversations about the support that would be in place for him and Kim. I cleared space in my diary to make regular home visits. During the next few days, I saw big changes in Kim's symptoms; at times she was lucid and at others very sedated. Kim's house was small; unfortunately, it had been necessary for her to be based upstairs, and she was asleep most of the time. She wasn't able to have her normal days in the lounge with the family. I have a strong memory of her sat next to me on the edge of the bed, with her head resting on my shoulder in silence and then asking, 'Carol, why do I have to die from cancer?' Often there is no sense to be made from tragedy, and acknowledging this was the most honest answer I could give to a young woman I had grown to understand and care for.

As Kim's physical and mental state deteriorated further, it got harder for Chris to cope; the community nurses who were dedicated to keeping Kim at home were becoming increasingly concerned, and telephone discussions were becoming much more frequent between all parties.

When this happens, and there are an increasing number of crisis calls out of hours, it is a clear sign of an impending carer breakdown. That was the background to three conversations that made it one of my hardest days.

Conversation 1 – a telephone call from Chris. Chris was very clear about no longer being able to cope: 'Carol, when you see your wife like this it makes you think differently. Everyone is thinking about what is best for Kim. Well, I am her husband, I am here with a 4-year-old boy, and when I see her covered in diarrhoea, screaming and fighting, confused, swearing and refusing to be cleaned, I know that this isn't best for Kim'.

Conversation 2 – telephone call from the community nurses, who agreed with Chris and had asked Kim if she would agree to be readmitted to the hospice. They told me of the gentle and indirect persuasion they had used with her, but she had refused. I asked to be put on the phone to Kim. I knew Kim well; I knew and considered all the views she had relating to this dilemma. The dialogue I chose to use with

Kim was short, very clear, and very direct; I considered (very carefully) that it had to be so. In my opinion, others were understandably shying away from giving Kim all the information needed on which to make a decision.

I started with: 'Kim, you know I have always tried to do what is best for you, given you the best advice?' I heard her mumble in agreement. I continued: 'Kim, Chris isn't coping, love, and this is going to get harder. I think it would be best if you came back in'.

There was a short silence before Kim answered, 'Then I have no choice'.

'Yes, you do, Kim, this is me being honest with you, and letting you make that choice', I assured her.

'I'll come in; it's best', she murmured.

Conversation 3 – with the doctor who works at the hospice 1 day a week (and hadn't been in the hospice for the last 3 weeks). 'Why is Kim coming back in, she wanted to die at home?' she asked me. 'That's so sad, after all that work, it was so important to her. When did you last see her, could it not have been sorted at home? She probably won't be that different than when she went home'.

The preceding stream of challenges and questions from the doctor took place in a room full of professionals, who all knew Kim and me. I could have cried; there and then, in front of junior staff, I could have cried.

The decision to persuade Kim (and I admit that I did persuade her) to be readmitted and use the words I had used was one of the hardest I have ever made in a career of 23 years. I responded thus: 'That decision was one of the most difficult I have ever made; I didn't reach it lightly. I did the best I could for the most people; I can justify it, should you want to discuss it further'. I honestly think that if the doctor had accused me of making an unethical decision, I would have made a much stronger response. I had led with my intellect but was acutely aware of my emotions.

I did cry afterwards; despite many words of understanding and support, I cried, and I cried for Kim. No one could remove my feeling of letting Kim down. That was between us; I knew that this was not what Kim wanted. I also knew from intellect and experience that what a patient wants can change, when circumstances change, in a way it would have been impossible for them to imagine when they made the initial decision. I knew I couldn't please everyone, and I sought to maximise the benefit for the most people. A truly consequentialist approach. When I look back, given the chance again, I would have done the same thing.

If, on reflection, that is your conclusion, having jumped through the emotional loops and considered everything, then it is as good as it gets in these dreadful circumstances, because some things can never be okay. I think I was brave too: no one else within that situation was going to make the decision; all three parties were looking to me for guidance, to take the lead and handle the difficult communication required.

A major influence on my decision, and one of the biggest learning points, was her husband's comments relating to everyone doing what we perceived to be 'best for the patient'. When he described the reality and emphatically stated that this was not best for Kim, he made a valid point. As professionals, we often know more than the patient, of what can go wrong and how hard it can/will be. Kim was increasingly symptomatic and the clinical signs were worrying, and that is the first part of my title: CLINICAL nurse specialist. Anyone can do whatever the patient wants, that would be easy. Sometimes it's so difficult to make a decision, and it costs, it costs emotionally.

Kim's death wasn't easy: she was young, fighting and struggling with noisy secretions. The hospice nurses found it harrowing. Had she been left at home any longer, I am sure there would have been a crisis admission instead of the admission calmly arranged and discussed. It wasn't what Kim wanted, and I have to reconcile my own guilt about that: I own that guilt, that I can feel it, consider it, and most importantly learn from it is vital. When I consider the principle of autonomy, I think of Kim's case. Because people matter, I would like to think that, if she were here, she would still lift her arms to be hugged because she felt safe with me.

Autonomy is the right of self-governance; it is a right of competent adults to be able to make important decisions defining their own lives for themselves. Kim's case raises many issues that are valid to communication in palliative care. Some of the professionals in the hospice obviously felt that she had the right to insist that she stay at home despite the concerns of her community nurses and family. It is difficult to determine at what point a patient is no longer the best person to know what is in his best interests. Kim's husband made a very strong statement about the stressful situation that Kim was in not being in her best interests. As Kim was agitated and (in her husband's view) confused, would her decision to stay at home now cause more harm than good, and was she still functioning well enough cognitively to decide? Should a person be allowed to impose their wishes on others when it adversely affects those others? Surely Chris has a right to autonomy too. Kant discusses the principle of autonomy as the ability to exercise self-restraint in choices, which affect others.[2] This is the problem when someone claims a right: it imposes a responsibility on others to uphold it, despite their wish being sometimes detrimental to others. Autonomy as a principle does not have intrinsic veracity. It is a concept that is applied and usually upheld in a very complex clinical arena.

Carol was clearly influenced by her past experience and knew that it was possible that Kim did not know what was best for her, now she was in circumstances that she had never encountered or envisaged. She was brave and set clear objectives for her discussion with Kim and stated clearly that the situation would get worse and that Chris wasn't coping. Kim hadn't considered either of these issues and in light of this information agreed to admission. It would not have been possible for Kim to make an informed decision without that conversation. As the expert, or the professional most experienced in having these discussions, Carol bravely led the conversation and crucially gave Kim clear information. By their own admission, the community nurses would have struggled to do this. They had (understandably) adopted a softer approach, using dialogue that wasn't clear enough for Kim to realise the true facts of the situation. Chris, Kim's husband, was distraught; the situation needed honest but brief dialogue. Kim clearly wasn't well enough for a subtle, long conversation which would gradually outline the reality. It is likely, given the clinical signs, that she would have fallen asleep mid-conversation, which would only have added to the stress of the dilemma.

Carol must have developed a relationship of trust with the community nurses, in the way she communicates with them, for them to have faith in her judgement, to hand the situation over to her and to be guided by the outcome. Palliative care professionals usually work well in teams, where they communicate effectively between different disciplines. The confidence that Carol herself must have had in those community nurses is evidenced by how she trusted their assessment of the situation at home, alongside listening to and respecting Chris's point of view. Carol clearly describes the tension between considering those views, her own assessment and the emotional burden of the long-held contract she felt that she had made with Kim.

It is those tensions that made these conversations so difficult for her. It is clear that the hospice doctor made the mistake of reacting only to the first level of knowledge. This is never helpful when assessing a palliative care patient. Clinical situations are often complex, and all the professionals who knew Kim expected this. The challenge made to Carol about her decision showed a lack of clinical insight and respect for how difficult the decision must have been for her. Interprofessional communication can be difficult, sometimes to the point of creating huge stress. It's important to be honest about that fact. It seems the doctor didn't see or acknowledge the emotion, tension, or complexities of the decision Carol had to make. Carol's short and clear answer was the most appropriate. She outlined the difficulties, offered insight into how she felt, stated why she made the decision, and made it clear that further conversation would take place in private. It's no wonder that this interaction might just have made Carol cry. She must have been mentally exhausted by the time that conversation took place. It was wrong of the doctor to not think beyond the first level of knowledge (that Kim was to be readmitted) and not consider both the reasons for this and the obvious complexities. It would have been decent of the doctor to acknowledge this after Kim's harrowing death, which needed to take place in an environment that supported everyone.

Kim's case and Carol's story illustrate well the tensions that can arise by always using patient autonomy as 'the trump card'. For any theory on autonomy to have true integrity and be plausible, it must distinguish between the general point or value of autonomy, and its consequences for a particular person on a particular occasion.[3] In this case, the principle of autonomy was overridden by the principle of beneficence.

Collusion

The issue of collusion is both challenging and common within specialist palliative care. Interestingly, the *Oxford Dictionary* places this word between the words *colloquy* (conversation) and *collywobbles*. This contextualises the problem well: it's about saying the right thing to the right person at the right time, and knowing when to do so can be anxiety-provoking for the professional involved.

The patient is the professional's primary responsibility. The feelings of the family, although valid and extremely important, are of secondary rank. The family/carers are usually the people who care about and know the patient the best of all.

JAN'S STORY

I'm a nurse and a daughter. My dad is my best friend and my world; we are close, and we talk about everything; we always have, even before Mum died. I know him, and I know how nurses can be too.

I have learnt that they can be wary of the daughter and the nurse, and I have seen them decide (with a measure of arrogance, in my view) to take up the role of advocate for the patient (without being asked) to protect the patient from the daughter who is a healthcare professional. I know this from years of experience, I know this is sometimes the case. I also knew clinically that it was highly likely that my dad's lung cancer had spread to his brain. He had deteriorated rapidly in the last few weeks, had lost so much weight, and was really overwhelmed with fatigue. So when I arrived to find him pleasantly muddled, with his cardigan fastened up wrong, I just knew. I got him sorted and sat with him; he was smiling at me, a smile that said, 'I'm weary, Jan'. It was Tuesday, the day the community nurse called. I didn't know which one it would be or how much cancer knowledge she would have or how she would handle the conversations about what was obvious to me.

Pat arrived, clearly busy (as community nurses always are). She was shocked at how Dad had changed in the week since she had seen him, and she felt a doctor's call was needed. She was right, and she was kind; I was glad of that and followed her out to chat. 'Pat, I'm a nurse too, and it's obvious that the cancer has spread to the brain now. Dad will need steroids, I am sure, but he doesn't need to know about the spread; it won't help him at all. He is 83 years old, unfit for radiotherapy, and he really wouldn't cope with any investigations or the worry. Would you pass on my concerns to the doctor before he comes to see Dad? I know my dad, and I will be here to help him'. The effects of my request were obvious immediately, as though I had thrust her into a huge ethical dilemma, a serious situation. For me, it was neither; it wasn't difficult to see that Dad's life expectancy was too short to endure scans and radiotherapy. He wouldn't live long enough to benefit, and chances were it would have made his symptoms worse. I knew that from both instinct and experience, and I could tell that the community nurse did not know this; she was unsure and worried that I was making decisions for my dad. Thankfully, she showed that she had heard and understood my request, and I could tell that she would keep to her word and have a talk with the doctor before he arrived. When she had gone, I worried about how I would be represented to the doctor: Would I be portrayed as the pushy daughter? The situation was distressing enough without me having to worry about this as well. But it's human nature. The nurse didn't know me, she had a job to do, and my dad was her first priority.

I understood that and respected it, but I was anxious about Dad and about what the doctor would say.

When the doctor arrived, it was Chris, one of the GPs that my dad knew well, and I had met him many times when I had taken Mum and Dad to see him. He gave me a warm smile as he came into the house (that mattered enormously). 'Now then, Ted, how are you feeling?' he asked Dad.

'Buggered', replied Dad. 'Absolutely buggered'.

'Let's have a look then, Ted', said Chris. He examined Dad's chest and performed a mini mental and neurological examination. It was clear that Dad hadn't passed either. 'Ted, I'm going to put you on some more tablets', said Chris.

'Not more bloody tablets; I'll be rattling', complained Dad.

Chris smiled and explained that they were only small and that they would make a difference, so it was important that Dad took them and that he would talk to Dad's consultant at the hospital. Typical of his generation, Dad accepted the advice. He would do as the doctor said; he always did, after moaning about taking more tablets.

'Well, don't give me anything to keep me alive any longer, I've had enough now, 83 years is long enough, and I'm buggered, Chris'.

As an experienced family doctor, I could see that Chris wasn't daunted by this remark. 'I won't, Ted, and I'll be back in a few days to check up on you'. They shook hands as Chris left, and I followed him outside.

He gave me the most understanding of looks, bless him. 'You are right, Jan. I am sure he has brain secondaries now, and he isn't fit for any treatment, so there is no point investigating. The response to steroids will be fairly diagnostic anyway, and I'll check with the chest physicians. It might be best if we just keep him at home with you and stop the outpatient appointments now; it's such a trial for him, and he is too weary to be waiting in the clinics. I will ring you when I have spoken to them'.

I thanked him warmly; he had taken so much pressure off me.

'I wasn't being bossy, Chris, but I knew it wouldn't help Dad to know what we were thinking', I explained. 'Oh I know, Jan; there is no benefit to telling him stuff he isn't asking about. You know if he asks me anything I will answer honestly and carefully, but I am not going to give information that he isn't asking for when we know it will probably just upset him further; it's not necessary or kind. Don't worry, Jan; he is lucky to have you. Are you okay?'

I assured him I was and thanked him again before going back to Dad, who was cheered up because Chris had been; he liked Chris.

'Good lad he is, Jan', said Dad. 'A right good lad'.

I could only smile and agree.

Specialist palliative care is always going to be both complex and complicated at times. There will often be ethical dilemmas and times when agreeing with the family to not offer information that hasn't been asked for is the right thing to do. Jan's story and the decisions made by Chris the doctor show this well. It can be arrogant of professionals to assume that they know more about what is best for the patient or know them better. It can be extremely hard for the relative who is also a professional. Including them in the decisions, listening to them, and treating them as the ally are crucial. Families have enough to cope with without fearing what a professional may say next.

The community nurse clearly listened to Jan and communicated effectively with the doctor, and the doctor displayed 'good old common sense' and medical friendship. He obviously trusted Jan's opinion, clearly due to watching her care for both her parents so well over the years. The time for a professional to be anxious about taking advice from the family is when all the evidence is to the contrary, when they see something that 'makes their antenna flash' as a warning that something isn't right in the family dynamics. Protecting the patient from the family should not be the default position for the professional. Assessing with accuracy, thoughtfulness, and care should be. Chris displayed warm and effective communication with Ted throughout his assessment and it matched the manner and generational style of the patient perfectly. However, within the informal interaction, Chris was making accurate clinical decisions based on the burdens and benefits of further investigations and treatment for Ted. He explained the rationale for this diagnosis and prognosis clearly to Jan and promised to communicate with the consultants involved in Ted's care. Clinical communication was shared amongst all relevant people. Most importantly, the appropriate treatment was prescribed, and part of that prescription was excellent communication skills.

Whilst Jan's story presents a typical example of collusion, it doesn't describe a difficult dilemma. Not all issues relating to collusion are so simple. This explains why the rules need to be.

Truth should always be the first intention of the professional. Offering information that hasn't been requested and isn't clinically required may cause unnecessary distress and harm to the patient and those who love them. The sentence 'Please don't tell him' can be translated to 'Please don't hurt him'. Applying kindness and common sense when listening and considering this request is very important. However, there will inevitably be times when it is necessary to inform the patient of clinical changes, even when he hasn't requested it or when the relatives have requested he not be told. For example, if a patient has to understand and consent to treatment, whether this is chemotherapy, wearing a neck support, or amending his behaviour to limit potential damage, he must be informed of all the facts. It would be impossible for a patient to embark on a toxic regimen of chemotherapy without having had his diagnosis and the objectives and side effects of treatment thoroughly explained to him. Also, a patient cannot be expected to follow clinical guidance if he does not understand the need for those changes or guidance. As a given, professionals should always explain the consequences of unhelpful collusion. Families, although knowledgeable of their own experience, do not have the wealth of experiences which professionals possess. Sharing this experience is vital; it is part of the professionals' responsibility to guide those in their care. It is good professional behaviour, because the professional has been in these situations before, she can see what can go wrong and how damaging the consequences can be. Whilst the situation a family finds itself in is very personal to them, the professional may have seen this situation hundreds of times. Having the courage to point this fact out to the patient or family at the time of making a distressing decision can be very helpful. When family members are in the midst of a personally distressing situation, it can be difficult for them to think about future events and to consider the effects of incomplete communication. Families are usually grateful when a professional shares the benefit of her experiences and allows them to consider issues beyond their cognisance.

All ethical decisions rest on the argument of burdens versus benefits. In the case study outlined, the GP had clearly assessed this. The important points are these:

- The first duty of care of the professional is to the patient and to tell the truth. If a patient is asking for information, there is no dilemma – the professional must answer honestly and clearly. If there are sound clinical reasons why a patient needs information, it is the professional's duty to provide it.

- If a patient is not asking and there is no clinical need to give more information, the professional can make the decision based on the burdens and benefits argument not to give further information. Telling the truth or, conversely, choosing to not give information when it is neither requested nor needed may, in time, be the decision that a bereaved family is the most thankful for. It can be the thing which they remember most clearly from all their sad experiences.

Futility of Treatment

Medical treatment decisions are the responsibility of doctors. They have the science, knowledge and expertise to make these decisions. The patient and their family do not. There may have been times when the patient was given information with which to make a choice relating to a type of treatment, but when it comes to stopping a futile treatment or not embarking on one, such as cardiopulmonary resuscitation (CPR), this decision rests firmly with the clinician in charge of the patient's care.

The exponential increase in modern treatments, the publicity afforded them by the media, and the rise of the concept of patient choice have made these decisions even more difficult for clinicians. It is, however, vital that the burden of choice is removed from the patient and his family.

The success rate for CPR, even within the acute setting where all supportive technology is available, is still only 17%. The original intention of CPR was for it to be used only in specific clinical situations, namely, to restart the heart in cases of, for example, drowning, electric shock, or heart attack. It has now become the default position in all deaths, where a DNACPR order is in place.

The discussion should be approached using a gentle but firm style. It is, of course, ethical to discuss these clinical decisions with the patient and family, if possible, but it is not always mandatory. There will be times when the patient is too weak or distressed to have a discussion relating to CPR. In these circumstances, the decision should be made and gently explained to the family. A choice should not be given to the family; it is a huge burden to give someone who lacks the science and knowledge to make that decision. The family's frame of reference is likely to be television programmes, where the success rate of CPR is an unrealistic 80%. It is unfair for them to feel that they are giving up on their loved one and impossible for them to turn down what they consider to be a chance of life.

The context for this book is palliative care only, and within this context, the success rate for CPR is 0%. There is no cure for being dead, for dying naturally from a disease. It is so important that the professionals involved in a patient's end-of-life care plan avoid the distress of futile CPR, which would be carried out if the appropriate documentation is not completed to prevent this happening. In the light of understanding the preceding, patients and their families are often relieved that there has been clear discussion and documentation relating to DNACPR. CPR is a violent act, sometimes necessary, and often successful, in other clinical scenarios. However, it can cause significant trauma at what should be a peaceful death for the patient and can create a dreadful memory for his loved ones. It is important that the professionals use clear language when discussing CPR, such as 'We know that you will die from this disease, and when you die, we will do everything we can to enable your death to be peaceful. We will not embark on treatments that won't help such as trying to restart your heart, when it stops'. Again, this concentrates on what will be done, rather than what won't be done. It also makes it clear that the decision has been made and a question hasn't been posed.

If required, the clinician (and there may also be a nurse involved in the discussion) may need to promote understanding by altering the patient's frame of reference with the appropriate use of medical facts. This information can change the way people think, quickly and usefully. They often have no idea that CPR would not work for a palliative care patient who had just died from his disease. It is the doctor's decision, and patients and their families should never be made to think that it is theirs. That would be both cruel and unhelpful. This discussion can be daunting for generalists and specialist teams should be contacted for support when needed. They are the experts in this field and acknowledge that guidance is often needed. Thankfully, the guidance published for clinicians is much less ambiguous and more helpful than it used to be. It is a medical kindness to be clear; it shows careful consideration of the facts and removes responsibility from those who are in the worst of situations. It can, of course, be extremely difficult to stop or refuse to start a treatment that the patient or his family is requesting or demanding. This book does not seek to underestimate that fact but to acknowledge it and encourage simple guidance in the face of complex emotions.

Whilst patients have the right to refuse treatment, they do not have the right to demand any, particularly that which a clinician considers to be futile. Families (except for lasting power of attorney – proxy decision-makers) do not have the right to refuse or demand a treatment for a patient. There are times when this has to be stated and times when the patient's or family's surprise and anger have to be managed.

In an environment of increasing choice and information giving, the patient and his family may be shocked to discover that a lot of decisions relating to treatment are not theirs. The clinician calculates the burdens and benefits of any treatment carefully. That she also communicates them well is mandatory. When patients and their families understand that a new treatment or further treatment is likely to make them worse, not better, it is easier for them to accept the clinician's decision. They often would not know this unless the clinician clearly explained it. Having had this explanation, if the patient or his family remains unhappy, the clinician can only acknowledge their feelings and offer further explanation or support, if needed. This may entail supporting the patient's right to a second opinion.

Once a professional has assessed the clinical situation carefully, used their knowledge to make a decision, communicated their decision kindly to relevant parties, and documented their decision clearly for the benefit of other professionals involved, they have done the best they can do. Professionals are responsible only for their decisions, not for the personalities and reactions of everyone in their care. They provide a professional service, not a personal relationship. It is a hard task and one which they do to the best of their ability in often very difficult circumstances.

Discussing Euthanasia

As the title suggests, this section relates to how to discuss euthanasia, when requested to do so. It is not about the ethics of whether euthanasia should or should not be legal. For this reason, the advice is simpler than may be assumed and follows on from discussions relating to futility. Again, a patient or his family has no right to demand a specific treatment from a clinician. Euthanasia is illegal in Great Britain – a clinician is not duty-bound to carry out any intervention that she feels may shorten the patient's life. It may be necessary to say this if euthanasia is requested and, equally importantly, to document the conversation in the patient's medical records. Should a patient or his family feel strongly about seeking euthanasia in a different country, a professional is barred by her professional code of conduct from providing this information. It would be the responsibility of the patient or the family themselves, irrespective of the personal views of the professional. The legal situation is clear and can be repeated clearly when required. There is no ethical dilemma here.

However, the challenge may lie in discussing with a patient and his family why they feel that euthanasia is their best option. It is valuable to ask that question, to enquire about their reasons for asking about euthanasia. There may be myths that can be dispelled and fears that can be allayed by understanding the principles of good palliative care. Knowing that effective symptom management, comfort measures and not using futile treatments are at the core of good palliative care may alter a patient's or his family's perspective regarding euthanasia. They may be unnecessarily worried that life, and in their view suffering, will be prolonged.

Describing the effects of an illness and how the symptoms can be managed is an essential part of the professional's role for palliative care patients. Explaining the value of medicines and clearly stating that professionals will aim to relieve symptoms as someone dies, and will not hasten death, may also be needed.

All patients have a right to their views and value systems; it is not professional behaviour to judge them, but a patient does not have the right to demand that a professional act unlawfully or intervene clinically when they consider it to be futile or harmful to the patient. The principle of autonomy applies equally to the professional and the patient. Once a person demands a right, it imposes a responsibility on someone else to uphold this right. Within the context of euthanasia, or futile treatments, a professional should be clear about not having responsibility to meet the patient's demand.

I believe that the subject of euthanasia is one for society as a whole to consider. Any change in the law would need careful consideration; the practical and judicial challenges are immense. Palliative care as a specialist area has a responsibility to enhance and maintain the quality of life of patients and their families and show the need for hospice and palliative care services worldwide.

Truth Telling

Truth should always be the professional's first intention. Most healthcare interactions involve simple truth telling. Therefore, a discussion on how to simply provide the truth isn't required. However, specialist palliative care is by definition complex, and professionals can regularly be faced with a complex ethical issue relating to how to communicate.

The truth can be both a kindness and a weapon. It can be both necessary and unwarranted. Whether to tell the truth or not is sometimes not simple. The following two case studies illustrate clearly why hard and fast rules cannot always be applied. They illustrate the difficulties that can present themselves to professionals.

BILL'S STORY

I've known Jack for many years. Recently, he presented with an increased problem passing urine; a physical examination revealed an enlarged prostate, not unusual at his age; he is 76 years old. The routine blood test revealed a high level of prostate-specific antigen (PSA). This can indicate a malignancy, and certainly it needs further investigation to exclude or confirm this. My problem is this: I know Jack is going away for the weekend. I also know he has fixed his mind on the PSA result and is worried that a raised level will definitely mean that he has cancer. I have just received a message from the receptionist to say that Jack has rung for his results, just before he goes away for the weekend. I have decided to tell him that the results are not back, and I can justify this to myself. There is absolutely no point in ruining his weekend. Nothing can happen before Monday when I will arrange the next investigations and talk to Jack personally, explain properly, and reassure him face-to-face. It doesn't fit into some textbooks, but I am his doctor, and I know I am right on this.

MARY'S STORY

Laura had recently been diagnosed with an awful cancer that isn't responsive to any treatment. She is young, aged 48 years, and is married to the most solution-orientated man I have ever met. He has been unable to accept that there is no helpful treatment in the UK and has arranged for Laura to travel to a South American country for a trial that entails administering a very toxic plant substance. This treatment is illegal in most countries, and it will cost the family many thousands of pounds. Laura is mum to a young family of two teenagers. I heard that she was seen by the oncologist and informed that chemotherapy wouldn't help. As she had her own plans, she accepted this calmly. She didn't ask questions; she has a strong faith and believes that prayer will cure her. I was also told that the oncologist did not discuss life expectancy with her but, as she left the room, expressed concern to the attending nurse that the patient and her husband had mentioned 5 years and as a doctor she expected it to be only weeks.

I was horrified! Here was a mum of two teenagers who was planning to leave them and embark on dangerous treatment who didn't know how precious time was for her. I felt burdened as a professional because I knew something that the patient needed to know and had an ethical right to know. I didn't make a quick decision. I knew better than that, and I didn't rush in. I discussed my decision with experienced colleagues. However, I did make the decision to make time to talk to Laura, and I had every intention of telling her the whole truth if needed. I felt so strongly that she was making the biggest decision of her short life without the benefit of having the full facts. So I asked Laura when she was planning her trip; I was reassured when she told me that it was planned for a few months' time. Sadly, I knew that she would have died by then. Furthermore, I asked whether she would change her mind about travelling if she felt unwell at that point and whether she would want instead to spend that precious time with her family. I was reassured that she had thought of this and had made the decision that if she felt unwell, she wanted to stay with her family. That was all I needed to hear; I had no reason then to give information that she wasn't asking for, but had I felt it ethically necessary, I would have. It had troubled me so much. The oncologist had 'bottled it', and I thought that was unethical. I know the consultation had not covered any details or time scales relating to the trip, although the patient had told the consultant of her plans.

The consultant hadn't asked any questions and crucially had not given the patient the full facts to enable her to make an informed decision.

It shouldn't be my job to 'mop up' the communication failings of other professionals, but when you work in palliative care, this happens. It becomes your problem when you know about it. I had a responsibility to tell the truth to Laura if needed and I would have. I knew the level of regret and distress that would have been felt by the patient and her family, and I couldn't just stand by and let that happen. My conversation took place 1 week ago, 2 days after Laura had seen the oncologist, and yesterday I admitted Laura to the hospice to die. I sincerely hope that the family can get back the thousands they have spent on travel arrangements in the 2 days since they saw the consultant.

Both case studies illustrate well how serious the issue of truth telling can be, and each provides true examples of how both truth and deceit can occur in professional communication. This chapter relates to communication when a professional is faced with difficult ethical issues and when tensions arise between the principle of veracity and the desire to protect the patient from the harm that truth may cause. Information, and, in particular, choices, can be a burden to patients who rely on professional recommendations. Both professionals made difficult and brave decisions in the patient's best interests. None of them made those decisions lightly.

Bill actually chose to lie, for what he decided was the patient's best interests. Whether lying is worse than withholding the truth is, of course, open to ethical debate. He clearly felt that there was no benefit in Jack being told of the raised PSA just before his weekend away. He demonstrated consequentialist ethics and chose to act in a way that maximises the good for the most people. *Primum non nocere*, 'First, do no harm', was an essential principle of Hippocrates's medicine. Bill's actions can be described as benevolent deception; perhaps because he knows Jack and his value system well, he has decided that Jack would trust his judgement more than his honesty. Had he taken a deontologist's approach, he would have told the truth because to lie is wrong and cannot be justified.

Mary found herself in a much more serious position. She obviously and understandably struggled with the crucial information which she felt Laura needed. She was concerned that Laura's decision to travel was made without fully understanding how this could impact on her and her family. The effect on her teenage children's grieving process could have been disastrous. Mary's decision again seemed consequentialist; it doesn't appear to be deontological. She doesn't rage against what the consultant has said but against the consequences of not providing Laura with the information she needed when she was fully aware of Laura's plans. Hippocratic medicine also asserts: 'Declare the past, diagnose the present, and foretell the future'. Mary clearly felt that the oncologist had shirked her professional responsibility, and she therefore took on that responsibility herself. In this case, the ethical burden of decision-making was passed to someone else. It was impressive how Mary negotiated how much information was needed.

The timescale of Laura's trip and the fact that she had made the decision not to travel if she felt unwell meant that Mary had no need to offer more information to Laura. These simple questions relieved the tension of the ethical dilemma Mary faced. Had Laura wanted more information, she would have asked for it. Whilst this situation was complex, it was solved by a simple, open, kind approach.

A recurring theme throughout this chapter has been the debate of burdens versus benefits. It's an issue that healthcare professionals have within teams and themselves on a daily basis. The complexity, challenges, and achievements regarding both the decisions and how they are made often go unacknowledged. It is difficult work but work that relies on simple rules.

It helps not to react to the first level of knowledge, to find out more, and obtain the facts. Ethical decisions within palliative care are rarely emergencies. It is vital to make time to consider and discuss these decisions. No one works in isolation; no one needs to. There are times when healthcare professionals pressure themselves to answer all questions and answer them quicker than they need to. There will be times when the most honest answer is 'I don't know'. Acknowledging how difficult the situation is for someone is usually the most helpful thing a professional can do when faced with a patient and a family in what is likely to be the worst of times for them. Suggesting and allowing time to consider a difficult dilemma is entirely appropriate. It is not defeatist; it is not avoidance; it is the opposite. It shows that the professional has taken the issues seriously and intends to deal with them respectfully and thoroughly. Palliative care will always take place in an emotionally charged environment; there will always be difficult ethical decisions. This chapter has sought to acknowledge and discuss some of those key issues in an honest and simple way. The acquisition and development of skills are a professional's responsibility; however, their experience, instinct, and kindness will be of equal benefit to those in their care.

> TIP: *The accumulation of evidence will lead you to see things that you haven't been formally taught.*

References

1. Beauchamp T, Childress J. *Principles of biomedical ethics*, 4th ed. New York: Oxford University Press; 1994. p. 454.
2. Kant I. *Grounding for the metaphysics of morals*, 3rd ed. Indianapolis: Hackett; 1993. p. 30.
3. Dworkin R. Life past reason. In: *Bioethics: An anthology*. Oxford: Blackwell Publishing; 1999. p. 308.

10

The Specifics of Advance Care Planning

I have a deep sense of change within, and of a permanently closer companionship with death.
– George Eliot on her 50th birthday

Hospitals are noisy, busy places in which to die. Privacy, despite professionals' best efforts, can be hard to achieve. Complaints to hospitals sometimes relate to end-of-life care and, in particular, to poor communication. More patients are choosing to die at home. The *End of Life Care Strategy* in the UK encourages communication regarding preferred place of care and death early in the patient's illness. The emphasis is firmly placed on advance care planning (ACP); a statement of wishes and preferences, it is not legally binding.

Discussing ACP is best undertaken by a skilled professional and should include open discussion to elicit a patient's wishes, recording his preferences, and sharing this information with all concerned parties. ACP also provides an opportunity for the patient's mental capacity (to make decisions) to be assessed and recorded and for the patient to record his wishes before his cognitive function deteriorates. An Advance Decision to Refuse Treatment (ADRT) document can be used. This is a specific recording of refusal of treatment in a pre-defined future situation (treatment can be refused, not requested). Providing certain criteria are met, this document is legally binding and only comes into effect when a patient loses capacity. A patient is judged to be mentally competent until proved otherwise.

Recording a patient's wishes is an important element of the existing legal framework, the Mental Capacity Act, which came fully into force in October 2007. The Act extends the ways in which people can plan ahead and set out in advance what they would like to happen should they be unable to make decisions about their care in the future. A patient may also choose to appoint a lasting power of attorney to protect his personal welfare. Mental capacity can be regularly tested; a patient may have the capacity for simple decisions but not for complex ones, and because illness is dynamic, capacity may fluctuate and will need to be monitored carefully and recorded appropriately. It is vital that any formal plans or decisions completed are witnessed, and that all relevant carers and professionals know of their existence. An ACP discussion allows an opportunity for the patient to identify his personal needs and preferences with professionals who can support them. The resultant document should be shared with every service which will be involved in supporting the patient so that they are aware of his priorities. His preferences and choices will be considered and accommodated, whenever possible.

Promoting and facilitating discussions about end-of-life care has many benefits, such as ensuring that wishes regarding organ donation after death can be raised with relatives who will ultimately have to give consent and that people have the chance to discuss their wishes about their funeral with relatives. It allows people to write or amend their will or

DOI: 10.1201/9781003427377-10

for same-sex partners to consider the validity of the status of their relationship so that professionals do not exclude them from involvement in their partner's care.

There will never be one single time at which it is right to initiate discussions about end-of-life issues, and it should not be assumed that the person would not raise the subject himself. For many people, this will be an interactive process. The process may start even before patients have a life-threatening illness, perhaps with their GP or community nurse, after a loved one has died.

When caring for a patient with a chronic illness, a point may be reached at which it becomes obvious that the patient will die from his disease. It can, however, be difficult to prognosticate accurately. Several prognostication tools exist, but one of the most useful is for the professional to ask herself 'the surprise question': 'Would I be surprised if this patient died within the next 12 months?' If the answer is 'no', then it is time to consider other questions, such as who will discuss end-of-life care with this patient, how will the plans be recorded and with whom? There are multiple triggers for this discussion, and these may involve changes in both social and clinical circumstances.

ANTHONY'S STORY

I loved visiting Edna. Even though she was 97 years old, she still had the twinkle in her eyes of a young girl who once danced with abandonment. She was always smartly dressed, complete with matching earrings. She kept her room at the nursing home tidy and surrounded herself with all her favourite things. She had often talked about her sadness at not being able to have children and she had survived her five siblings. This had contributed to her independent and private nature. We had often had very open discussions about her failing health and she was aware that her kidneys and liver 'weren't working as well as they used to'.

When I arrived at the home, I could see immediately that Edna was pensive. She greeted me warmly and asked with interest about my family; she had remembered everything about our previous conversation. We chatted for a while and then she paused. 'What are you thinking about, Edna?' I asked.

'Oh, I'm really upset today, Anthony', she answered. 'Mary, who was next door, was taken into hospital last night but she didn't want to go. I have just heard that she died when she got there. It's awful. Oh, it has upset me, I knew Mary well'.

I could see that Edna was really upset and waited until she spoke again.

'I don't want to go in hospital again, Anthony, I want to be here at the end'.

I held her frail hand and spoke gently: 'Edna, I'm so sorry that happened to your friend. We can talk about what you want and write it down so the same thing won't happen to you, if you like?'

Edna looked up and spoke very quietly, 'But the nurses will ring an ambulance. When I asked them about Mary and told them how much she dreaded the hospital, they said they had to ring an ambulance!'

I could see that Edna felt she had no control over the situation and a worried expression had replaced her peaceful one. I started to reassure her by saying, 'Edna, there are many things we can do. First, we can make it clear to everyone looking after you that you want to stay here, at the end, and not go to hospital'. I explained further: 'If you had a nasty infection or there was treatment that we thought would help you, we could ask you about it, and if you wanted to go just for treatment, I could arrange it and arrange for you to come home quickly'. I paused while Edna considered my words. 'We won't be sending you in hospital for no reason, Edna', I continued. 'We can fill out some forms today, and I will talk to the nurses here and your doctor so that everyone knows the plan. Don't worry, Edna, we can do this your way'. She listened hard as I continued. 'We won't let anyone do things that won't help. When you are at the end, we will keep you here and keep you peaceful; for ladies your age, it wouldn't be kind to try and resuscitate. An ambulance won't be needed, Edna. I will do a form that will stop anyone trying to do that', I assured her.

'Can you?' Edna asked. 'Really?'

'Yes I can, we will do it together, and I will ask one of the nurses to join us too'.

It didn't take long to fill in the documents needed and to explain them to the nurse looking after Edna. She had heard of such documentation but had never used it. Both Edna and the nurse looked pleased when I left, and I really felt I had done a decent job that day.

Patients in both residential and nursing homes can be particularly vulnerable to unnecessary ambulance calls and CPR. This is often due to the owner's fear of litigation. Good, clear planning and documentation can easily resolve such problems. That Anthony took the opportunity to educate the nurse was very valuable. Many healthcare professionals want to do 'the right thing' and don't know how. As the expert in end-of-life care, Anthony took an opportunity and used it well. Many patients and nurses in care home settings would benefit from end-of-life care planning and education.

In conclusion, it is helpful for professionals to consider instigating discussions regarding a patient's preferences and wishes for care during his illness and death when they realise that the patient's life expectancy is likely to be less than 12 months or when the patient has raised concerns that relate to this issue. Whilst for specialist palliative care professionals this may include most of their caseload, these discussions do not always have to take place immediately or during a single visit to the patient. Using the following phrases can help the discussion:

- It is important that I understand what is important to you; can you tell me the things that matter to you?
- It is important that I write your wishes down, so all the professionals involved in your care are aware. Is that okay with you?
- When you are unwell where would you like to be cared for?
- You seem like a man who wants to stay at home; would you want to stay at home at the end of your illness?

If a patient lacks capacity, due to illness or unconsciousness, it is crucial that the professional has a clear and empathetic discussion with any family present. Together with the family, the professional can then act in the patient's best interests.

Discuss and record the patient's wishes when possible. When appropriate include the family.

Always consider the changes to circumstances and be prepared to check whether the patient's wishes have changed. A patient may have initially stated a wish to die at home, but at the end of life, he may have changed his mind and request admission to an inpatient setting.

> **TIP: *Making plans for a death does not cause anyone to die quicker, but it does help them to die on their own terms.***

98% of people wanted to know they were dying. 60% of doctors didn't want to tell them. 60% of people knew it anyway.

(Elisabeth Kübler-Ross, *On Death and Dying*)

11

Breaking Bad News within Palliative Care

Bad news is just that; it can't be made into good news.

The key word regarding breaking bad news is *negotiation*, a theme that follows on from what was discussed in relation to the issue of collusion.

This chapter does not outline any particular model; rather, it discusses the key issues and skills that are needed to break bad news well. It also has its emphasis firmly on the scenarios typical to palliative care and respects that the initial diagnosis of a disease may already have been given by another skilled professional.

Breaking Bad News: Patient or Family

The news may need to be broken to the patient or to the family. If it relates to the patient's medical situation, the patient should hear the information before the family; it is his moral right and the duty of the professional. To give information to anyone before the competent patient without the patient's permission is unethical and a breach of any professional's code of conduct.

Bad news may therefore be broken to the patient and then the family or to the patient and his family at the same time, with the patient's consent. Family within this context relates to the person or persons chosen by the patient.

Who Breaks Bad News?

There is no law that states that bad news has to be broken by a doctor. However, it often makes clinical sense for the doctor to have this conversation because the patient and his family may have questions relating to treatment, which only a senior doctor may be able to answer. She may, therefore, be the best person to have this difficult discussion. The advent of multidisciplinary work has greatly influenced who breaks bad news. Often senior nurses or clinical nurse specialists have all the necessary information and skills to perform this task well.

The issues to consider are Who has the high level of skill needed? The closest relationship with the patient? What information needs to be relayed? Where is the patient? Is he in

DOI: 10.1201/9781003427377-11

hospital or at home, and if the latter, is he physically fit to come to a hospital clinic? Therefore, the decision of who breaks bad news must be carefully considered. It is also often the case that professionals in the community, the patient's GP or community nurse, know him best and are well placed to have these discussions.

Where to Break Bad News

Where to break bad news is an important consideration: the ideal situation of a purpose-built room, however, cannot always be met. The 'how' is always far more important than the 'where'. Patients only remember the 'where' when the 'how' was traumatic. Palliative care professionals come at the end of a patient's illness journey and often listen to a history of poor communication, including statements such as 'He stood there with his hand on the door handle' or 'We were taken into a small green room'. Conversely, statements like 'He was so kind; he told us so gently' or 'Even though he was so busy on the ward round, he made time for us' are also heard. It's not the 'where' but the 'how' that is remembered. Bad news can be broken well in a busy corridor or badly in a quiet room with lamps, tissues, and potpourri.

The purpose-built room has its drawbacks, especially for patients who have endured lots of hospital treatments and have sadly become familiar with the ways in which these teams and wards work. The walk to 'the special room' or the appearance of a nurse in the consultation room can send its own messages. Within the hospital domain, communicating information with such messages is often unavoidable, but it is still worth considering an alternative. It can be argued that the outpatient setting is a better place than the ward round in which to break bad news. As a hospital inpatient, the very fact of being attired in nightclothes can alter one's confidence level and behaviour, and privacy is unavoidably limited due to the close proximity of other patients and staff. The medical 'posse' of the consultant and several junior doctors is familiar and clinically necessary whereas, in the outpatient or GP setting, the clinician has dedicated time specifically for the patient, who is feeling more himself in his normal clothes, and privacy is much easier to maintain.

Difficult discussions often take place in the patient's home and for the clinical reasons already mentioned, and relevant in palliative care patients, such as failing health and mobility, this is often kinder, more practical, and therefore more appropriate.

Face-to-Face or By Telephone

There will be occasions when a professional may have to consider whether to break bad news over the telephone. Local policies and specific circumstances will inevitably dictate the action taken. For example, if the death was expected, a family member may have already stated that they do not want to be contacted during the night and are content to be informed in the morning. This will have been agreed in advance. If the death hadn't been expected 'quite so soon', but the family were aware that the patient was in the final phase, the professional may still feel it is appropriate to tell the family of the patient's death by telephone, particularly if the family live some distance away.

SUSAN'S STORY: BREAKING BAD NEWS BY TELEPHONE

'Mrs Clarke, it's Susan, the nurse from the ward.

'I was just going to ring to see how he is.'

'I'm afraid he became very unwell this morning. Is your son with you?'

'Oh dear! Yes, Paul has just arrived; we were just going to set off'.

'I'm so sorry, Mrs Clarke, Eddie became very unwell rather suddenly this morning, and he died a few minutes ago'.

Pause. Allow reaction.

'Oh dear God, oh no' (as Mrs Clarke cries and tells her son, amidst tears).

'Mrs Clarke, Eddie died quickly and peacefully, and he wasn't alone. I was with him, and I will look after him until you get here. Take your time; he is not alone'.

Pause.

'Are you all right, Mrs Clarke? It's still a shock, even though we knew it was the end'.

'Oh dear, poor Eddie'.

'Can I have a word with Paul?'

'Yes, love, I'll put him on. Paul, Susan wants a word'.

'I'm so sorry, Paul, it happened so quickly; your dad was very peaceful. I've just explained to Mum that you should take your time – we are with Dad. I didn't want you to be rushing up the motorway'.

'I'm glad you told us because we would have. We'll just get ourselves together and set off'.

'See you when you get here; just take your time, he is in good hands'.

It is easy to see the kindness and common sense that influenced Susan's decision. It is also important to note that Susan knew Mrs Clarke and would have carefully assessed the burdens and benefits of this decision. Within the context of caring for the dying, such decisions are common, yet they are carefully made for the best of reasons. It would have been natural for Eddie's family to rush to be there at the time of death; had they rushed and arrived to discover that Eddie had been dead at the time of the phone call, it may have seemed cruel to them. Susan's style of talking about Eddie as a person to be cared for rather than a dead body showed respect and thoughtfulness. Although clinically, Eddie was now 'deceased', for Mrs Clarke and Paul, he was still a person. Undertakers adopt the same lovely approach when dealing with loved ones and it matters enormously.

Cues

There are clinical imperatives that dictate the ways in which hospitals and clinics function, and many are unavoidable within the context of breaking bad news. The message here is for professionals to be aware of the cues given to the patient. These cues may include the title on a professional's badge, such as clinical nurse specialist, Macmillan nurse, or the name of a hospice. A professional can only take mental note, and acknowledge to themselves, that these subtle ways of communicating information exist within the environments that they take for granted. Whilst professionals are busy with their tasks and the art and science of their jobs, their patients and their families are sensitive to all the information around them and are often trying to make sense of a situation which is anxiety-provoking. A clear introduction or a kind and gentle look will go a long way to dispel fears. A patient will know that a professional can't change the facts or the clinical arena but that she will deal with him kindly, and it is this that is remembered amongst all other messages given.

Breaking bad news within palliative care can relate to various issues that alter the patient's expectations of his future in a negative way. For example, at initial diagnosis, evidence of recurrence, stopping active treatment, and the inability to work, maintain nutrition, mobility or sexual function. Furthermore, what represents bad news to one patient may, strangely, be a relief to another. The range of normal reactions is wide.

How to Break Bad News

Having acknowledged the 'who', 'where' and 'what' of breaking bad news, we now concentrate on the most important issue: 'how' to do it.

There are many helpful models for professionals to use as guidance. The crucial fact is that breaking bad news relates to skills, not rooms or models. The latter exist as valuable educational guides. Good manners and kindness are pivotal issues in this area of communication.

Kindness is just as much about body language as the spoken word. An open posture, a gentle voice, and a kind expression say more than words ever can. Patients can tell whether a professional has time for them or not, the signs of being busy are obvious, and it is so important that a professional considers and hides these impressions.

Sitting down to give bad news is essential; it gives the impression that a professional has time (which she often hasn't got much of) to listen and talk. Troubles are very heavy things, too heavy to be lifted up; it's much easier for a patient or his carer to pour them out when the professional is sitting. Sitting on the floor, on the edge of the bed, a chair, anywhere, if possible, helps and has a huge effect on how the patient copes with and remembers the discussion. For professionals working in the community, removing their coat on arrival at the patient's house also sends a strong message of having time for the patient. Making a patient feel as though he is the only one in the professional's care is an art, and the way of achieving this can involve such simple acts.

Planning to Break Bad News

Planning is important in all areas of clinical care. When breaking bad news, it is crucial. Planning within this context relates to the professional having all the necessary facts and knowing who else the patient would like to be present during the discussion. This preparation is vital and should also include the professional eliciting the following information from the patient: what is already understood and how much information is wanted.

When it is difficult to assess those issues, direct questions may be needed, such as 'How do you think things are going at the moment?' or 'In your situation, patients are often wondering about …'. Or to state the difficulty openly and clearly, for example, 'Everyone is different – some patients at one end want to know everything, and some want to know things on a need-to-know basis or only when they ask. It would help me if you told me what kind of person you are and how you would prefer me to give information to you'. Patients usually respond clearly to this question and offer guidance to the professional that also sets the framework for how they will communicate in the future. This is especially useful to a professional who is in the position of breaking bad news to a patient that she is meeting for the first time.

Given the complexity of a patient's clinical problems, the expertise of another specialty may be needed. Such open and respectful discussions also allow the professional to set other boundaries, such as stating that she will always answer a patient's questions honestly and ask for the patient's permission to discuss his case with his family if requested to do so. The first point offers a warning to the patient that whenever he asks a question, he will be told the truth, and in light of this knowledge, the patient can choose not to ask questions, which may elicit answers that he is not ready to hear.

The second point can save the professional a lot of time in the future and, from the outset, enables her to understand the patient's value system relating to communication within his family group.

Having established the patient's understanding and information needs, the professional should break the news slowly and clearly, using non-ambiguous language. What may be obvious to the professional has often not occurred to the patient; the term *heart failure* is an example of this. Sadly, palliative care relates to the care of patients who have a life-threatening disease, by definition a disease that will progress and from which they will die. They will die, not pass away, lose a fight or go to sleep. Palliative care demands quite rightly that the professionals involved can cope with those facts and discuss them gently, clearly, and openly when required to do so.

A patient's choices and those of his family can be greatly influenced if bad news is delivered well. For example, a will may have to be made or adjusted, a holiday or wedding may no longer be possible or may need to be brought forward. The list of changes and complexities within any family is endless. A professional can never alter the facts or stop the emotional reaction to bad news. Her role is merely to give the information that is requested and needed so that the patient and his family can make their own choices and cope better than they would have without knowing all the facts.

JOANNA'S STORY: NATURAL SKILLS

I have been a specialist nurse for many years, and I am now enjoying watching my daughter as she progresses as a junior qualified nurse through her nursing career. She is determined not to work in palliative care, she tells me regularly, as she regales me with tales from the wards, as I used to do with my mum. I had to smile at the following conversation. 'You know, Mum, today we had a lady who was dying, and her daughter was sat with her all day. Her dad is already dead, and she is alone with three small kids. She was asking me what to do, whether to stay or sort out care for her kids. It was obvious her mum was dying. I felt so sorry for her, so I asked one of the doctors, who knew her mum, to go and answer her questions, so she could sort things out for her kids and stay with her mum. When he came out of the room, I asked what he had said. He told me that when she had asked if her mum was dying, he had told her that everyone dies. Okay? he said and started to walk away!!! No!! I said, "It's not okay; it's your job to tell her the truth that she is asking for, so she can do the right thing. She needs your guidance and kindness, it's your job, so I shall stand here blocking your path, until you go back in there and do your job and then it will be okay"'.

I smiled at her, which elicited the response, 'I'm not going into palliative care; I'm not like you'. Oh yes you are, I thought.

Joanna's daughter is young; a more mature experienced professional would no doubt have been a little more polite but would hopefully have been just as firm in challenging bad communication, the effects of which have drastic short- and long-term consequences for patients and their families. It is not uncommon within palliative care for professionals to be in a position of trying to undo the damage done by previous poor communication.

JAMES'S STORY: BREAKING BAD NEWS WELL

Sometimes I feel as though I spend all day with bad news, carrying case notes under my arm. Today was one of those days. Gerald was a typical, lovely old chap, a life-long smoker who called 'a spade a spade' kind of chap. I had liked him and his sons from the outset. I had suspected the worst from his symptoms; the results of all his investigations merely confirmed my concerns. Gerald wasn't my first bad-news session in clinic, but it would be the first time I would deliver bad news to Gerald.

'Hello, Gerald, you are looking rather smart today'. I welcomed him into the consultation room and guided him and his two sons into the room. The lung cancer nurse helped them settle into seats and smiled warmly at them. 'I'm Katie', she said. 'I'm one of the specialist nurses, I work with Dr Davies'.

Gerald smiled back and shook her hand.

'How are you feeling, Gerald?' I asked first.

'Weary' was the first word he replied. 'Weary and I've lost my appetite, the weight is falling off me, and my lads are pestering me to eat, and I can't face it at all'.

'That's not unusual, Gerald; we can talk about that later. How is your breathing?' I asked.

'Not too good sometimes. I soon get out of breath, especially going upstairs', he added.

'Mmm, you seem a little breathless now, Gerald; let's have a listen to your chest'. I stood up to examine Gerald. He followed all my requests to the letter, trying really hard to pass what he saw as a test, inhaling and exhaling with care and gusto. 'I have all your results back, Gerald, including the bronchoscopy, and your symptoms don't surprise me. It's not good news, I'm afraid. The mass we talked about on your X-ray is definitely cancer, and it has spread to your liver'. I waited for the information to sink in, and watched the family of three exchange looks, as though they had dreaded this but, in the light of this information, were still lost for words.

There was a few minutes' silence, and I allowed this to pass before I spoke again. 'Could you tell me how you are feeling, Gerald?' I asked gently.

'I did suspect, Doctor, because you had warned me when you saw the X-ray, and I knew something was wrong. Do I have to have chemotherapy? I'm not too keen on that idea, to be honest. Bill had that, and it made him worse'.

'I'm sorry, Gerald, this is serious. It's a large cancerous mass and chemotherapy may be helpful; it could help enormously with your symptoms', I answered and waited again while they exchanged looks.

'I have thought about it, Doctor, and I won't have any chemotherapy. My family and I agree; it's an absolute no to chemotherapy. You can't say for definite that it will give me more time, can you?' he asked.

'No, Gerald, I can't', I answered honestly. 'It may do, but I can't guarantee that, no. But, as I say, it may help you to feel better by reducing the breathlessness', I added.

'I really don't want it, Doctor, thank you', he repeated. 'I know you are all doing your best, but I really don't want it'.

I allowed the silence; it was clear that Gerald was thinking of what to say. He looked up, met my eyes, and asked me, 'Is it worth me buying new shoes, Doc?'

I smiled in return. I knew what this meant but knew from experience that it was wise to check. 'Gerald, if you want new shoes, you should buy some and enjoy them. Are you asking me how long you have to live? Some patients want to know, and some patients would rather live each day as it comes. I will answer your questions honestly', I assured him.

'I like it straight, Doc, I want to know how long', he added clearly. I decided that he had given me a clear instruction and that a clear answer was appropriate.

'In my experience, Gerald, you have a few months. It's impossible for me to know exactly, Gerald'.

'Thanks, Doc, I like to know, you see, so I can get sorted', he said.

'Gerald, my advice is to get your affairs sorted and then forget about them, no one dies quicker because they have done a will. I've done mine. Getting that sorted will be on your mind until it's out of the way. Knowing exactly when you will die doesn't change anything really, Gerald, once you have got sorted, as you say. From there, it's about enjoying life as much as you can, time with your sons, and getting out in those new shoes', I advised.

Gerald's sons remained quiet but attentive. Their body language was not questioning, and their focus was on their dad, not me. I decided to speak to Gerald again. 'Gerald, a lot of people in your position are wondering how they will feel, as time moves on. Is there anything you are wondering about?'

'Yes', said Gerald, 'What will happen now; will I be in pain?'

I smiled back at Gerald as I explained, 'Gerald, I don't know the answer to everything, and I can't say exactly how you will feel, but I do know what commonly happens. As I explain, I will tell you what we can do about it; this conversation is about what we can and will do. The air isn't going into your right lung as well as it should, which is why you feel breathless, Gerald, and before you leave, I'm going to prescribe some medicine that will help with your breathing. The nurse will talk to you about this afterwards. Feeling weary is normal; it is part of this illness, and you will find as time goes by that you need to rest more.

You will notice that what you could do last month is harder now. You will see the changes, and it'll be gradual, Gerald, as though those new shoes you are going to buy are getting heavier. Katie will talk to you about this as well; there are ways of conserving your energy, some helpful tips. Eating small and often is the key; losing your appetite is part of the illness; big meals won't help. Eat just what you fancy and eat little and often if you can. Pain isn't usually a problem, Gerald; if you do have any pain, your GP and community nurse will be able to help you. Katie will talk to them to let them know about our chat today, and if there are any problems, they can ring her, and she will talk to me. If your breathing does get much worse or if you start to cough up more, let Katie know, radiotherapy could help. It isn't like chemotherapy. It's an X-ray treatment, easily done, and it can often help a lot. Gerald, it's important to remember that there are things we can do, and medicines and people that will help'.

I paused to allow them to take in the information. 'Katie is going to take you next door to explain things further and have a chat and you will be able to ask questions. Is there anything you want to ask me?'

Gerald rubbed his chin and answered, 'I don't think so, Doc, thanks for telling me the truth. Will I be seeing you again?'

'Yes', I assured him. 'Katie will sort your appointment and the prescription for the medicine to help with your breathing'. As Gerald seemed satisfied, I turned to his sons and asked if they had any questions.

'Will he be all right going to the club for a pint? He loves to do that', his son asked.

I smiled back and answered, 'I insist he does, for as long as he can. Live life as normally as possible, Gerald. Katie will take you next door'. We shook hands as they thanked me and left.

It's impossible to feel good about breaking bad news. I have learnt that if I can look back and decide that I couldn't have done it any better, then I have done it well.

James's story displays the key elements of breaking bad news well. He was well prepared, having acquired all the facts, and established how much Gerald wanted to know, and he allowed him to express his feelings. Within all the models and guidance, those are the two key issues of breaking bad news. Furthermore, he used clear language and talked about cancer and dying. He used his clinical experience and expertise to pre-empt and encourage questions from the patient and his family.

It was Gerald and his sons who chose the style and pace of the consultation, yet James still did his medical assessment and reached his clinical objectives within the consultation. Gerald left with all the relevant information, having had his questions answered and the opportunity to talk further about what would happen next and how he would be supported.

The use of silence was clear: when a patient or his family is silent, they are usually thinking of what to say next, framing their questions. It can be hard for professionals to get used to this, especially when breaking bad news; the temptation is to say something kind or helpful, but it helps more to allow the patient and his family to adjust to what has been said and choose their questions or to allow them to verbalise their feelings.

The important issue was how well James negotiated the discussion with Gerald. This relationship first began at an earlier meeting, when James had discussed the earlier abnormal X-ray. James had obviously intimated at that visit that the mass seen on the X-ray may be a cancer, and a 'warning shot' had therefore been given at this time.

James remained clinically focused and concentrated the bulk of the consultation on what could be done rather than what couldn't be done. This is the essence of communication in palliative care, discussing what can be done at a time when the patient and his family are feeling that there is nothing more that can be done.

Possible Challenges

There are times when the issues of collusion and breaking bad news collide: when the patient requests that other family members are not told. It is of course his right to make this decision, but for professionals with experience of the possible consequences of this action, it is important to intervene and explain the implications of withholding information in this way.

Children can be a difficult issue for parents to deal with, and often their instinct is to protect them for as long as possible. When they are struggling to cope with their own emotions, dealing with the emotions of others seems impossible and may be avoided by collusion. Parents may not realise how not telling their children will affect them. It is vital that children are given honest, simple answers when they ask questions. It is not necessary to give small children information they haven't asked for. When something doesn't make sense, they will ask a question. Explaining why Mummy is in hospital, for example, will often be necessary. The most important issue is that children of all ages are aware that doctors and hospitals can sometimes make people better but that sometimes they can't. This helps prepare them for two very important issues in life. Knowing that sometimes sick people cannot be cured prepares them for the subsequent sad discussions that may have to take place. However, knowing that illness can be cured or managed will reassure them, especially when someone else in their world becomes ill. The parents can refer them back to this conversation. Children who have experienced the death of a close relative or friend can be very afraid that everyone who gets ill or who develops cancer will die. It is very important that they understand that this isn't always the outcome.

The teenage children of a dying parent in particular need honest clear information. They may already be self-absorbed as they struggle to make the natural transition from childhood to adulthood. All parents know that teenagers do this by pulling away from them, that they can seem detached and hard to reach as they live between the worlds of a child who needs support and the self-sufficiency of adulthood. These can be confusing and difficult times for the whole family and the world of an adolescent may have to be interrupted by having a clear conversation forced on them. They can be so concerned with themselves that they appear selfish and uncaring, and their persistence in this behaviour must therefore be challenged clearly when needed. Most teenagers will be very engaged with a deteriorating situation and this confrontation may not be necessary, but when parents or siblings avoid open discussions with an adolescent in the family, it is vital that the professional points out the long-term consequences of this behaviour for the adolescent. When an adolescent is unaware of the real situation, they are unable to modify their behaviour which can cause guilt in the bereavement phase. It can be very damaging to them psychologically; they deserve the truth, and any collusion should be firmly challenged by the professional.

Having these discussions is very difficult for the parents, but they are the best people to have them. They will need guidance and support to do this. The professional can direct them to this guidance either verbally by giving them written information or by directing them to useful websites. It is important that the professional makes herself available for further discussion either with the teenager or their parents. This is likely to be one of the hardest discussions that a parent will ever have; if they are aware of how critical it is for their children's future well-being, it will help them carry out this heart-breaking task and allow them to realise that protecting their children from the difficult truth is not in their best interests. The professional can give examples of bereaved teenagers they have seen who are resentful of the fact that they weren't made aware of the severity of the situation or were excluded from it. Time is impossible to get back. The most a professional can do is to give the right information at the right time to the right people, enabling them to make their own choices based on the real facts.

CHRISTINE'S STORY

I thought I knew what to expect from the visit to Tim and his wife, Shirley. I was wrong! Tim had had lymphoma for 9 years and was dying imminently from secondary leukaemia. He had told me that he suspected this during my last visit. He also requested that his fears be confirmed for the sake of him and his family. He wanted to make plans for the rest of his life and both he and Shirley wanted to have clear discussions with their family. They had two teenage grandchildren and one of their daughters was expecting a baby in 3 months.

Having had a long supportive discussion about this during my first visit, I had decided to talk to their consultant haematologist before she saw them in clinic the day after as it seemed appropriate that I pass on their request for a clear prognosis. I had made a subsequent appointment with Tim and Shirley to support them after that consultation. I was therefore amazed that they (in their words) were no wiser. From the dialogue they had quoted me about their consultation, I couldn't understand why their clear questions hadn't been answered. Asking whether he would see his grandchild born in 3 months seemed a clear question. I was surprised that the consultant told them that she was 'hopeful' (when just 2 days ago, she had told me she felt his life expectancy was now weeks and that she would tell him this).

They were so disappointed and clearly desperate for guidance. I hadn't expected this, but I knew I had to tell them the truth.

'Tim, I can see you have thought about this, what length of time is going through your mind?' I asked.

'Weeks', he replied. 'I'm going downhill by the day and I just want to know', he replied as he sat looking down and wringing his hands.

Shirley added, 'We can see it; every day, he is weaker, we just need to know. We want to take the kids to our caravan while we can; we have family stuff to sort out'.

I waited for Tim to raise his head and give me eye contact. 'I'm sad to say that you are right, Tim', I told him. 'Time is short for you now and it is likely to be only weeks, how many, I can't be certain, but you are right to sort the family stuff'. I waited during their silence and watched the looks that passed between them. They already knew, there were no tears. They almost looked relieved.

'Right', said Tim. 'We know where we are now, sadly'.

'I'm so sorry this has happened to you', I said to them both.

Tim was quick to answer. 'It's okay; we know now, so we can get sorted; we knew anyway'. 'Why couldn't the consultant have told us that?' Shirley asked. 'We asked often enough, if you can tell us, why couldn't she?'

'Maybe she felt it would be easier for you to chat about it at home as she knew I was coming', I offered, as an explanation.

Afterwards, we had a long chat about where Tim wanted to die. I had already arranged for the necessary forms and medicines to be in the home, so I updated the GP and community nurses about the conversation I had had with Tim and of Tim's wishes. It was a sad visit but not too difficult, and it didn't take long. At their request, I spoke to their haematology consultant to inform her of my conversation and to tell her that they had decided not to attend her clinic again. She was grateful for the first point and agreed with the second. It wasn't a difficult conversation; some things don't need to be said, but some things do! I know it's not easy to break bad news, but someone had to for the sake of Tim and Shirley. Obviously, the consultant had decided to leave that to me, but it would have been helpful if she had told me that before I visited!

The possible complexities within communication extend to those that take place between professionals, as well as those involving the patient and his family. Christine's story makes this point well. She is obviously an experienced professional, undaunted by the task that she unexpectedly faced that day. It is prudent to point out that Christine already had all the clinical information that she needed and that the patient wanted to be told with his wife present. Both Tim and Shirley made it obvious that they already knew the prognosis. Christine's task was merely to confirm their fears; whilst this task was sad, it was also simple. Christine could have taken issue with the consultant for not answering Tim's and Shirley's clear questions as previously agreed and for not informing her that she hadn't had the agreed conversation. It would have allowed Christine to prepare; after all, she had been professional and considerate enough to give valuable information to the consultant to allow her to prepare to deliver bad news.

Part of Christine's wisdom is shown in the fact that she accepted easily that this could happen and didn't react strongly to the consultant afterwards. It isn't unusual for one professional to have to assume the responsibility of delivering information when another professional has chosen not to. Maybe the consultant had felt that she was too 'overloaded' with work in the clinic that day, perhaps she just didn't feel she had the necessary rapport with the patient, and it is even possible that the conversation hadn't been exactly as Tim and Shirley said it had. The 'why 'of it obviously wasn't the priority for Christine. She accepted the problem and offered the solution. Her agenda was to support the patient by giving the clear information that was needed. The fact that she ended her discussion with Tim and Shirley with good care planning was so important. In addition, she communicated quickly and effectively with all the professionals concerned, without criticising those she would need to maintain a good relationship with.

> **TIP: Be prepared, have all the facts, and decide who needs to be there.**
> Elicit what the patient already knows and how much they want to know. Allow the ventilation of feelings.
> If the preceding are remembered, the professional breaking bad news won't go far wrong.

12

The Dying Phase

Life is a sexually transmitted disease with a fatality rate of 100%.
– Anonymous

Everyone dies. Whether by worsening chronic disease until the body is unable to function, suddenly by trauma or by an acute event such as a heart attack, everyone dies, just once; there is no cure for being dead.

The dying phase has the potential to be the phase of care that is most vividly remembered by the family. Therefore, the importance of this phase of care being handled appropriately cannot be overestimated.

Dying in the 21st Century

In modern times, it is not unusual for people, even those who are middle-aged, to be death-naïve. For many, witnessing someone dying is both a new and scary experience. In recent times, dying has moved away from the home and into the hospital, so death has been removed from most people's experience. Current worldwide healthcare strategies seek to alter this.

It is, however, an imperative that all requests and all choices cannot always be met. The significant projected increase in the number of deaths that require palliative and end of life care. In the UK, approximately 600,000 people die every year on average, but by 2040, this number is expected to reach nearly 800,000.[1]

More and more people are also set to die with complex palliative care needs in the coming years due to the UK's ageing population and the increasing number of people living with more than one chronic condition. Fortunately, with the advent of hospital and community-based palliative care teams, the hospice philosophy has moved into all clinical arenas. Excellent care at the end of life is about skills and attitudes; it is not about buildings.

Within any clinical setting, it is crucial that the dying phase is identified and acknowledged. It is only when all professionals agree that the patient is dying that appropriate care can be planned and delivered. It is about 'changing gear'. This may include both stopping and starting treatments. It may be necessary for the professional to instigate discussions that lead to agreeing that the patient is dying. Hospital medical teams (within the acute sector) can often be so focused on a treatment agenda that the signs of deterioration are missed. It can be daunting for professionals to have discussions with clinicians when the objective is to stop treatment.

DOI: 10.1201/9781003427377-12

MANDY'S STORY: PROFESSIONAL CHALLENGES

My colleague (who was new to the role of specialist nurse) dreaded working with this particular consultant. It was always the same: too busy to talk and often seemed reluctant to stop treatments. I had met the patient that she was concerned about and his lovely wife. It was obvious that Don was dying and that the intravenous drip, copious medicines, and daily blood sugar monitoring weren't helping. In fact, they were making it harder for him. Norma, Don's wife, knew he was dying, and she hated the drips, tubes and 'constant messin', as she called it.

Dr Riley, Don's consultant, was a good doctor, a good man no doubt, but he was 'an island'; he seemed to work and think in isolation and could be very difficult to talk to; consequently, most nurses didn't try to. I have learnt simple techniques over the years, such as reminding the doctor that we share responsibility for end-of-life care; to be brief – doctors are too busy for protracted conversations. Even when professionals are just trying to be polite, doctors like brief, clear information. I have learnt not to write 'Janet and John stories' in the medical notes for the same reason. They won't be read, and professionals who take too long to make a point will be avoided. There are some professionals that we all hope will be on answer machine when we ring, so we can just leave the information in a message rather than be caught up in endless chit-chat relating to past events. In my view, clear, brief information is the most professional way to communicate (and we are all too busy to have our time wasted), and I am aware that it has taken years of experience to gain the confidence and skills I have today. I agreed to talk to Dr Riley about Don and take my new colleague with me.

As we entered the ward, I could see him, busy in the office with his junior colleagues around him as he scanned a patient's notes and muttered, it seemed, to himself. To be fair, that was probably how he concentrated. I had no doubt that this doctor cared about his practice enormously. He looked up at us and continued with the discussions with his team, so we waited. As he moved away, I stepped in his path, smiled warmly, and said, 'Dr Riley? I'm Mandy from the palliative care team – could you spare me a moment to discuss one of your patients – Don Clarke?' Although his chin stayed down and he didn't actually speak, his eyes came up to meet mine. I didn't waste time: 'I have just been in to see Don and his wife; he has deteriorated significantly, hasn't he?'

'I haven't been in yet', he answered, 'but his bloods are back …'. He began to flick through the notes, and I edged in next to him to look at the blood results. He ran through all the deranged values, muttering and thinking as he talked.

'Oh dear', I said. 'They are the bloods of a dying man, aren't they? That doesn't surprise me, and it won't surprise his wife'.

He nodded in agreement. It was that acknowledgement I had hoped for. So, I ventured in to meet my objectives, to encourage appropriate end-of-life care. 'He still has a drip up, Dr Riley, and daily blood sugars are being done. Can we stop that now? He is, as you say, in the dying phase, and the extra fluid is becoming a burden; he sounds wet-chested. His wife understands.

I have spent time with her; she is aware he is dying and wants only comfort measures now'. He turned to his junior staff to ask them to make the changes, and I went for my conclusion: 'Dr Riley, I know you are busy, so is it okay with you if I write suggestions in the patient's notes for your junior doctor, stopping non-essential medicines, some anticipatory drugs? Oh! And we do need the DNACPR confirmed, I have discussed it; his wife understands and agrees Don is semi-conscious now'.

'Yes, fine', he answered and he turned to his junior doctor: 'I'll leave that with you'. The junior doctor nodded in my direction. I stepped sideways to allow him to pass, gave him my best smile and said, 'Many thanks, Dr Riley'. He grunted a thank you and even smiled slightly. The whole conversation took about three minutes. It took much longer to write the plan properly in Don's notes:

> Discussed with Dr Riley – patient in dying phase. Please stop non-essential medicines, IVI and BMs.
>
> DNACPR needs confirming. All above discussed and agreed with wife. Suggest the following comfort meds, all S/C PRN:
>
> Diamorphine 2.5–5 mg
>
> Midazolam 2.5–5 mg
>
> Buscopan 20 mg
>
> Haloperidol 1.5–3 mg

Thank you for your help, ring me on Extension 5437 if needed. Mandy. Palliative care team.

I explained all the preceding to the nurse looking after Don. She was grateful, and I knew she would make sure that the junior doctor didn't forget. The bulk of my time was spent with Don's wife, explaining and reassuring her of the changes and, most of all, giving her time to talk about how she felt.

Mandy's story offers clear insight into common problems that can arise when working in hospital teams with dying patients. Crucially, the skills she used can be transferred to all settings, when talking to a busy GP, for example. She obviously set clear objectives and was able to reach them quickly. It is helpful to summarise the key learning points.

A clear introduction of self, polite acknowledgement of the consultant and of how busy he was, blocking his path, and stating that the conversation was about his patient were helpful. Professionals, as Mandy stated, share care. Her input would be both in the patient's and his wife's interests and in the consultant's interest, as Mandy was doing a specialist assessment and making appropriate recommendations. Her expertise saved the consultant and his team time, both in clinical decision-making and in terms of communication. Mandy allowed the consultant to adopt his style of management by focusing on the clinical facts, and she took this opportunity to join him as a colleague to discuss the recent blood results. She didn't wait at the side; she stepped forward as a professional with a shared interest in the scientific facts.

She took the cue of the deranged bloods to identify and agree that the patient was dying. Once that has been agreed, it is much easier to concentrate the discussion on appropriate care. Doctors respond well to clinical terms. Asking what phase of care the patient is in is always helpful; naming the phases curative, palliative or terminal can alter the doctor's perspective and clinical plan.

Once they had agreed that this was the dying phase, Mandy asked if she could work with the junior doctor to organise good end-of-life care. She briefly stated what was needed and that a supportive conversation had already taken place with his wife, which had included the DNACPR discussion. Importantly, she made it clear that written suggestions would be in the patient's notes. Equally valuable was the time she spent supporting Don's wife and her less experienced colleague. It is likely that Don's wife will always remember those discussions; how her feelings and opinions of how her husband's death should be supported, were heard, and acted on; and that she was comforted at such a distressing time. Mandy's colleague will have benefited from the example that she set. It is the theory being put into practice that will have helped so much. No doubt she will aspire to gain that level of confidence in how she communicates. Mandy perhaps made it look easy, but the maxim 'the harder you work, the easier it gets' is appropriate. It is said that an expert can be defined as someone 'who hides their mistakes well'. Even someone as skilled and experienced as Mandy will have made lots of mistakes and been nervous many times in her career.

End-of-life care discussion and plan, all done in three minutes, and Mandy saved the consultant and his team a lot of time and he knew it; she deserved his smile.

The plan was clearly written and communicated to all relevant professionals. The nurse on the ward needs to be fully informed of any plans to enable her to support the plan. The junior doctor may not be familiar with the medicines and doses used in palliative care, and he will be grateful for the clear guidance. It is highly likely that given the confident and helpful approach that Mandy used, the junior doctor will seek her advice again in the future. This will enable Mandy to build on the clinical relationship by supporting and educating others about quality end-of-life care.

It is easy to see how the roles of consultant and ward nurse can be substituted for those of the GP and community nurse. Communicating by mirroring styles is a useful tactic. If patients have a more informal style, then using that same style can be part of the introduction. The objectives when communicating about end-of-life care are the same: assess, set objectives, provide clear introduction of self and joint clinical agenda, agree on a plan, and communicate clearly in verbal and written form.

Death can be a very difficult issue for professionals to deal with; it is very sad and can pose complex problems requiring careful, considered judgements. That these challenges are dealt with openly and communicated effectively are the key factors in ensuring high quality at the end of life.

Integrated Care Pathways

There are integrated care pathways (ICP) that support the above agenda. An ICP is a tool which provides written guidance relating to a host of different clinical scenarios and outlines appropriate care. This includes stopping unhelpful and burdensome treatment and concentrating instead on comfort measures and supportive communication with carers. It is a multiprofessional tool that supports the whole team and replaces all other patient documentation. It provides an effective mechanism for monitoring and sustaining high-quality end of life care in all settings. The focus is on the management of symptoms, effective communication, and supporting the patient's spiritual needs.

The ICP should be carefully and sensitively outlined to the carers. Whilst it is acceptable for professionals to use the phrase 'care of the dying pathway' and various abbreviations amongst themselves, this language is too blunt to use with carers who face the loss of a loved one. Rather, it is kinder to discuss the plan as being an excellent way to provide the best possible care and *support the patient as they die.*

An ICP organises care for a well-defined group of patients at a well-defined time, namely the dying phase – the last few days of life. It does not apply to other patients in any other situations. The identification of dying is, as previously stated, essential if the right care is to be delivered. An ICP includes a clear list of questions for the assessing professional to support the diagnosis of dying. The decision is made by senior clinicians and agreed within the team. An ICP therefore promotes both knowledge and high-quality care. It neither hastens nor postpones death, it is only as good as the professionals using it and good communication is pivotal to its success. However, in the absence of such tools, the philosophy of good end-of-life care can still be applied, as Mandy's story illustrated. Mandy knew what her purpose was within that clinical situation; her priority was to instigate excellent end-of-life care by encouraging clarity, altering the treatment plan and communicating well.

All professionals in all settings can transfer the philosophy described by asking themselves the following questions.

- First, has dying been diagnosed and has the fact the patient is dying been understood by the patient (if appropriate), the family, and relevant clinicians?
- Does the family need further explanation or support?
- Have the objectives of care been set to maximise patient comfort and has spiritual support been considered and facilitated if desired?
- Is the plan understood and communicated to all relevant parties?
- Is it clearly understood that end-of-life care necessitates ongoing reassessments?

A Word About Syringe Drivers

It is important to be clear about the reasons for using a syringe driver in the dying phase. This may be explained to the patient during previous discussions regarding how the dying phase is managed. It may have been valuable to reassure the patient that the medicines he may require will be delivered in a different way when swallowing becomes too difficult. It is common for patients to be worried about their symptoms at the end of life. A simple explanation of the small unintrusive device is helpful. Knowing that a steady dose of medicines will be used to keep them comfortable and pain-free is very reassuring. It will prepare them for the changes in care that often take place.

It is crucial to have a clear conversation with the family when a syringe driver is used. Their impression may be that the patient died quickly when the syringe driver was started. The professional should state clearly that the syringe driver is being used because the patient is dying and is therefore unable to swallow the medicines that he needs. These may be medicines that are new to the patient and are needed to ensure comfort in the dying phase, or the same medicines that the patient was taking before he became unable to swallow. It may be necessary to be very clear and state that professionals relieve a patient's symptoms as they die, and the drugs used will not hasten death.

Communicating with and Supporting the Family

Earlier an outline of how to communicate and instigate appropriate end-of-life care was provided. It is valuable to concentrate a little on how to support the patient's loved ones at this time.

MANDY AND NORMA

Had I not met Norma before, the conversation would undoubtedly have been harder, but I had, and Norma was a gentle spirited lady, very open, and therefore very easy to talk to. I asked Norma to come with me to the 'quiet room' while the nurses attended to Don's personal care.

We held hands down the busy corridor. I could sense that this event was becoming a 'blur' to Norma. I tried to imagine being on a busy ward, with people you hardly know, while the most significant person in your life is dying. I think some things are beyond our imagination and most things we don't understand until they happen to us. It is understandable that some people adopt a child-like state when they are set amongst the busy, parental machine of a hospital. I sat for a while, just holding Norma's hand. I waited for her to speak; it was obvious, as I sat just watching her, that she had been collecting her thoughts.

'He is more peaceful now, I'm glad, he did seem so restless before. Will it be today, do you think?' she asked, as she stared at her hands and turned her wedding ring round and round.

I met her eyes to answer, in a gentle quiet voice, 'I think so, Norma, he is coming to the end now, and we will do everything we can to keep him comfortable'.

'Oh, I know', she assured me. 'Everyone has been so kind, wonderful, all of you; no one will criticise the health service to me'.

'Norma, do you want me to contact anyone for you? It can be hard sat alone, and you will be here for a good while yet', I asked.

'No, love, I don't think I do', she calmly answered. 'My daughter is on her way from America; we have talked about this time, and she will get here when she gets here. He went down so quickly, didn't he? She spoke to her dad yesterday, and she is okay. You see, with my daughter living in America, Don and me are used to being alone together. I don't think I want anyone else here, but thanks for asking. Does he know I'm here? I think he does, you know; he squeezes my hand sometimes. He always was a softie'. She paused to dab her eyes, with the lace-trimmed hankie. Everything about Norma was gentle and unassuming.

The sadness in these circumstances can be overwhelming, to be with a loving couple who have endured so much and to watch as they prepare to part is truly humbling. I could feel my eyes fill with tears as I answered, 'Norma, you chose a good one, didn't you?' She smiled a confident smile and nodded. I continued: 'Things did change very quickly for Don, that can happen, he will have been getting weaker gradually and things have just overwhelmed him now'. She was nodding in agreement as I spoke. 'You know, Don will still know that you are here, that's why he squeezes your hand. Keep talking quietly to him if you want to. You have been so close. I don't suppose there is anything left for you to say that Don doesn't already know. That's a success story, Norma'.

I allowed the silence as Norma considered my words. 'I will leave you to be with Don now, if you need anything or you have any questions, just ask the nurses, and if you want to talk to me, ask them to ring me. I will talk to you tomorrow anyway, Norma, and to your daughter. I am happy to explain anything and talk things through, if it helps'.

She nodded and continued to stare at her hands before she looked up, smiled, took a deep breath, and raised herself to her feet to go back to her husband and complete the last part of their journey. I was aware of composing myself as we walked hand in hand back to Don's room. I didn't speak as I hugged Norma, I didn't need to, but as I leant over Don I whispered, 'Your lovely lady is here, Don – all is well'.

I admit that I had tears pouring down my face as I left. The older generation are so impressive. They can be so grateful for little things, so accepting, and often not as fragile as we think they are. It was clear that Don and Norma had been through so much together, a real old-fashioned partnership, the 'thick and thin' that we talk of.

There was little left for Norma to say; she just needed to be there and to know that Don knew that she was there. For me, the real issue in terms of spirituality is helping a person or loved one to feel that their life had meaning, that they mattered, and acknowledging their successful marriage was my way of doing that. They deserved that acknowledgement. I wanted Norma to feel some pride in her sadness and know that we would be there, if she needed us. Beyond explaining the bureaucracy of death, I knew she wouldn't, though.

Mandy's description of the supportive discussion she had with Norma makes some important points. The humanness in her approach is evident. The discussion, led by Norma, was tailored to her personality and level of need. It was simple and reassuring, the gentleness in Mandy's style matching Norma's reactions. For Norma, these were inevitable; she accepted her impending loss and needed little further information. The fact that Mandy assured her that she was doing all the right things was probably all she wanted to know. Norma gave Mandy some cues: that her daughter hadn't been able to be there because of how quickly things had changed. Acknowledging and explaining this was very helpful. Offering ongoing support and realising that the daughter who hadn't been there may also need it showed both wisdom and kindness. Professionals cannot own the experience of those they care for; they can only share the experience, be in the same moment, be the one who can still 'think straight', and show that they care.

MICHELLE'S STORY

Today I am the worst nurse in the land! I have failed to be of any use at all. I have obviously got it all wrong and I tried so hard with this girl and her fiancé. I tried really hard. I have known Donna for a year, and it's been a horrendous one. She had a rare and horrible cancer. What has happened to her body shouldn't happen to anyone. It has been heartbreaking to watch, and I remember every time that she cried in my arms, like a little girl, sobbing at the cruelty of how her young life was being ruined. She was 22 years old. She was a newly qualified professional, with her future in front of her. Every setback and consultation, which involved more bad news, was devastating to her and her fiancé, Paul.

I had always planned my visits to coincide with their emotional reaction to these consultations. I admit that part of me, although truly sorry for Donna and Paul, felt some sympathy with the professionals I heard being berated so venomously by her. Anger and blame were always their initial response; it was understandable, and you can't expect people to accept the unacceptable. I was never able to achieve any change in the way they thought and reacted; they steadfastly believed that someone should be able to stop this happening. They seemed to cope by being angry, but it was damned hard work being on the receiving end all the time. It was both worrying and exhausting.

When I admitted Donna to the hospice for symptom management, it didn't surprise me that I was the one asked to have all the difficult conversations (well, me and my consultant colleague Ella, that is). I truly think that during that time, Donna and Paul grew to hate us; that's how it felt. Yet someone had to tell Paul not to go to work and that Donna was imminently dying. His refusal to accept that meant he was making choices that he would possibly regret later. I hated doing it, and I knew he hated me for it too, his anger was palpable, and he verbalised it well! But only to us! They were both lovely to all the other members of the team but visibly recoiled if Ella or I were within their sights. I picked up the cues and kept my distance whenever I wasn't needed.

When Donna died, one of the ward nurses asked if I would pop in and check that Paul was okay. I was reluctant, I admit it, but because he could be difficult to deal with, I felt I should comply with the request to support the staff. He visibly recoiled from me as soon as he saw me; 'No, Michelle, I don't want to see you', he said in front of all the family members, who hadn't met me before and turned to see who the enemy was. I know that sounds emotional, but it was emotional; it was horrible.

I can rationalise how they were angry with most professionals and certainly always angry with those who told them the awful truth in answer to their constant, reasonable questions. When I meet patients and carers like that, I am experienced enough to know that I too will be on the same blacklist sooner rather than later. I am happy that Ella and I practised kindly and ethically and that the situation would have been worse had we not been brave enough to have those conversations. I can even acknowledge that Paul could not and would not see it that way.

We were there as professionals, not friends. Yet two issues bothered me: I was clearly intensely disliked, which felt horrible, and that's human, I suppose. Whilst I am not there to be liked, when you are disliked so strongly when you are working hard to do the right thing, it hurts.

Second, I wondered whether I did the right thing for Donna in how I handled her emotions. I wondered whether fostering false hope would have helped her more. Paul needed to know not to go to work that day, and I am okay with that. But should I have constantly played the 'grim reaper' role with Donna, or should I have allowed her to rage against her illness and prognosis and fudge the truth when needed? I am struggling with that now. The textbooks are great, but in real life, sometimes you just feel like you got it wrong, despite your best efforts. The outcome here was wrong, and I feel like the worst nurse in the world today.

Not all communication goes well. There are times when professionals feel that they have failed, even after reflection, as Michelle's story shows. Sometimes it is very hard. The range of reactions is vast. The case studies highlight how different those reactions can be. Age may or may not be relevant. People are so different. Illness does not sanctify or improve anyone. In reality, it often exacerbates the characteristics that are already there. Paul clearly wanted solutions, answers, but only the kind he wanted to hear. Their coping mechanisms were totally different from those of Don and Norma.

Michelle had adopted and maintained the role of truth teller and supporter to the less experienced members in the team. This happens in specialist practice and within medicine. It takes knowledge, skill, and courage, yet it can also mean that as a person in a professional role, such difficult interactions come at a cost. It is possible that some patients and their families assume that professionals are hardened to their work in palliative care. They may reach this conclusion because of how well those professionals keep their composure and maintain their focus on clinical effectiveness. When faced with people like Donna and Paul, it was impossible for Michelle to get past the barriers they put up, to enable her to show a more human touch. She was unable to share their distress, because they rejected the facts that were causing it. When faced with the barrier of anger, the only thing that Michelle could do was to acknowledge their feelings and maintain professional integrity, by doing the right thing and telling the truth, when it was needed. Donna and Paul did not want to be closer to Michelle, and that was clearly hard for Michelle to accept on a personal level, and that's okay! Professionals are only human, and sometimes the communication they are involved with hurts.

Michelle's concerns may provoke a variety of responses in the reader. What is obvious is that Michelle is self-aware and still capable of worrying whether she got it right or not. For that reason, she will continue to learn, adjust, and improve her practice.

TIP: Be kind, confident, and clear in your communication. All three aspects will be valued and remembered.

Reference

1. Hospice UK, May 2022.

13

Assisted Dying

The Current Legal Situation

The subject of assisted dying is both complex and complicated, it is also dynamic. Assisted dying remains unlawful in the UK. Although in the UK and across the world legislation is constantly under review, numerous bills have passed through both houses of Parliament in the UK. The current assisted dying bill is awaiting further parliamentary processes and it proposes:

A bill to enable adults who are terminally ill to be provided at their request with specified assistance to end their own life; and for connected purposes. The terms of the bill follow.

For the purposes of this Act, a person is terminally ill if that person—

(a) has been diagnosed by a registered medical practitioner as having an inevitably progressive condition which cannot be reversed by treatment ('a terminal illness'); and

(b) as a consequence of that terminal illness, is reasonably expected to die within six months.

Treatment which only temporarily relieves the symptoms of an inevitably progressive condition is not to be regarded as treatment which can reverse that condition.

In terms of UK law, this chapter is accurate at the time of writing.

The Purpose of this Chapter

This chapter does not anchor itself in either moral attitudes or religious beliefs. It seeks only to help increase confidence in those who are both kind and brave enough to have these sensitive discussions. As the definitions used in this subject can be confusing, I have included a glossary of contemporary terms at the end of this chapter.

Part of education is always about provoking thought and debate. Any views expressed here are personal to me, and I have written within the scope of UK practice and law. I respect that your views and experiences may well differ. I do not put forward the rights and wrongs of this issue, but in order to be balanced and not sidestep pivotal issues, ethical dilemmas, and the political realities are discussed.

As a non-religious person, I hold the view that the sanctity of life issue has little relevance in the argument. Neither do I feel comfortable that most participants on panels where legislation is discussed express only their own strong religious convictions as their argument. I believe that non-believers and humanists should be included in the public

DOI: 10.1201/9781003427377-13

debate to fairly represent the populace. You will all have your own views, and I would encourage you in your research to study both sides of this debate, which continue socially, politically, and legally. You will find studies and information that reaffirm your views, whether they are for legalising assisted dying or against it.

It could be argued that every time someone claims a right to a particular treatment or procedure, a responsibility to deliver it is imposed on someone else. Most carers would not want to kill a loved one either directly or indirectly, and in my experience, most professionals feel the same way too.

If assisted dying is legalised in the UK, I feel that we can assume that the professionals involved will be both passionate and skilled in that area of practice.

The way forward in the debate is fraught with moral dilemmas and judicial challenges. It is not my intention to drown the reader in a moral swamp, as interesting as the subject and as varying as the views can be, so I refer to case studies which include examples and advice on how to communicate sensitively and clearly on this very important topic.

Every new high-profile case invokes huge coverage in our media. What isn't covered is the existing high volume of excellent end-of-life care that relieves the anxieties and suffering of the patients and families in our care. The coverage rarely discusses the need for timely end-of-life care planning, which in my view ameliorates many of the anxieties relating to the manner of our dying.

This chapter seeks to redress the balance, quash some myths, and help professionals encourage open discussions about dying and the importance of recording their preferences and choices. How we die is too important to be left to chance, and it often is, purely because our patients do not realise which choices they can make. And it is just as vital that they understand that some decisions, which for good reasons can only be made by the medical profession – such as stopping unhelpful treatments and/or making DNACPR decisions based on the futility of cardiopulmonary resuscitation at the end of life.

In all four nations of the UK, ReSPECT forms are used in clinical practice; ReSPECT stands for Recommended Summary Plan for Emergency Care and Treatment.[1] The ReSPECT process creates a summary of personalised recommendations for a person's clinical care in a future emergency in which they do not have the capacity to make or express choices.

Such emergencies may include death or cardiac arrest but are not limited to those events. The process is intended to respect both patient preferences and clinical judgement. The agreed realistic clinical recommendations that are recorded include a recommendation on whether CPR should be attempted if the person's heart and breathing stop.

Discussions with loved ones, when they exist, and with the patient's consent to do so, are mandatory for both these issues.

I acknowledge that this topic is highly emotionally charged and that those emotions are often fuelled by language such as 'unbearable suffering', which, interestingly, is never defined. No one, if asked, would agree that they want to die that way. As professionals, we know that there are additional options: clinically, administratively, legally, and practically.

It is crucial that professionals know what those options are so they are able to support people who want to discuss assisted dying. It's an important opportunity to listen, acknowledge, and guide people who rely on us. In fact, it's our professional responsibility to do it and to do it well; we can do no more.

I would assert that in healthcare where holism is seen as optimal, we have to keep focused clinically in our communication and stop short of taking responsibility for existential anxiety. Our role is to provide the best advice and to be a friendly clinician, not a personal friend.

The Clinical Landscape

Everyone is a product of their experiences, and we can't change those experiences, but we can educate patients and try to reframe their understanding of them when able to do so.

Armed with increased knowledge, they will be much more capable of making their own choices and will therefore increase the chance of having them considered and respected at the relevant time.

Whether you can support a patient's wish for assisted dying is easy to answer in the UK: you cannot; it is against UK law, and you risk prosecution. In countries where it is lawful, you will have clear processes to follow and safeguards to which you must adhere.

Between 1 April 2009 and 31 March 2023, there have been 182 cases referred to the Criminal Prosecution Service (CPS) by the police that have been recorded as assisted suicide. Of these 182 cases, CPS did not proceed with 125, and the police withdrew 35. At the time of writing (April 2023), 4 cases are outstanding.

The oft-referred-to British Social Attitudes Survey for Assisted Dying from 2017[2] states that 77% of people feel a person with a painful incurable disease should be able to legally request that a doctor end their life. It is important to acknowledge that many people see the practice of a physician's administering a lethal dose of drugs to end the life of someone who fits the above criteria as compassionate medicine.

In all honesty, throughout my decades of working in palliative care, only two patients have asked me to end their life. One asked directly for voluntary euthanasia, and one asked for assisted suicide, but perhaps most importantly it prompts the following question:

When actually faced with impending death, do many people really want to die or have their death hastened? And if not, why not?

There has to be a reason why so few have raised this issue with me. I have cared for people from diagnosis to death. Sometimes they met me at the very end of their lives and or in the last few months, but often I had been their clinical nurse specialist for years.

It was not uncommon for patients with non-malignant diseases or those with breast and ovarian cancer patients for me to have had a supportive if intermittent relationship with them over many years. I was the one they returned to every time there were new fears or they had been given bad news. My point here is that I did have trust and a rapport with my patients, and given that symptom control was my domain and what they relied on me for, I think I would have been the person that they would have chosen to ask about the possibility of assisted dying.

In my view, many people do believe that assisted suicide should be legalised, mainly because it is framed in the media as being a respectful way to stop 'unbearable suffering'. We never see articles in the media showing any data from answers to the following question, 'If you had a terminal illness and the professionals caring for both you and your loved ones gave you the confidence that they would, listen to and respect your wishes and ensure that you were as comfortable and pain-free as possible would you want them to end your life?' I assert that questions relating to assisted dying are not balanced and that is unhelpful when this subject is so important.

I can see why most of the professionals involved on the parliamentary panels have a background in specialist palliative care, as by definition most of their patients are going to die, but this should not be at the exclusion of other specialties.

The results of the survey carried out in 2021 by the British Medical Association (BMA)[3] demonstrate why avoiding bias in representation is so important. When asked whether they believed that the BMA should support a change in the law to permit doctors to prescribe life-ending drugs, the survey showed that members from the following specialties were more likely to agree that the BMA should support change:

- Otolaryngology (53% supportive)
- Clinical radiology (52%)
  - Trauma and orthopaedic surgery (52%)
- Anaesthetics (51%)
- Emergency medicine (50%)
- Histopathology (50%)
- Intensive care medicine (48%)
- Obstetrics and gynaecology (48%)

Conversely, members from the following specialties were more likely to believe that the BMA should oppose a change in the law:

- Palliative medicine (70% opposed)
- Clinical oncology (44%)
- Geriatric medicine (44%)
- General practice (39%)

I appreciate that if you are a clinician, you will have much more knowledge than the public, and you may even have thoughts of how you would feel if you were faced with certain diagnoses. It may even be that your profession mostly includes end-of-life care and is one of the professions most likely to be drawn on to actively participate in assisted-dying practices. End-of-life care clinical experience will have given you an extensive insight into the reality, away from media reports. You will be able to predict any logistical and practical issues and have a deep understanding of the anxieties experienced as and when someone dies. I understand that, and I feel it's that level of understanding and humanness that you can take to any discussions that you may face about assisted dying.

Practical Issues Demonstrated by Case Studies

For reasons of honesty and integrity, the following case studies relate to UK practice only.

ARTHUR'S STORY

Arthur had recently been admitted to the oncology unit with severe pain. He was 77 years old, married with 2 children and was a retired company director. His diagnosis was prostate cancer and an MRI on admission had revealed inoperable spinal metastases which had compressed his spinal cord.

He was non-compliant with his medicines, analgesics appropriately prescribed by the oncologists. He was both angry and demanding. This medical history made his case complex and appropriate for referral to Lynne's Specialist Palliative Care team in the hospital.

Lynne arrived on the ward, spoke to the doctor and nurse involved in his care, and read his case notes thoroughly. She was particularly interested in what had already been said to him. She needed to know what style of communication had been used, how he had reacted to it, and exactly what the treatment plan was. Even though she was hopefully bringing new ideas/possible solutions to the situation, she also saw her role as a way of demonstrating good teamwork with the referring team. This promotes confidence in the patient with our care.

Just as she was about to enter Arthur's room, there was shouting from Arthur's room and a nurse came out visibly upset. He had threatened to throw his lunch at her.

Now certainly wasn't the time to go in and see Arthur, but she could usefully listen to the nurse and offer her support, and she was keen to find out how his family felt about the situation.

She rang his wife, Vera, who was very upset and had been the recipient of his anger for a long time. He hadn't stopped being angry since diagnosis. Arthur had always been strong-willed and liked to be in control, and he had been a keen and accomplished sportsman. He could not accept any weakness or physical deficit. She was very apologetic for his bad behaviour and sounded utterly exhausted.

Lynne had left Arthur alone for half an hour and then went into his room. She introduced herself as a palliative care specialist nurse who worked with the medical oncology team and told him that she had been asked to see him about how they could better manage his awful pain.

Arthur immediately asked her for euthanasia. 'I'm not interested in tablets. I want euthanasia; will you do euthanasia?'

She explained clearly that she was unable to do that but would like to understand why he felt that way.

Arthur roared, 'I have a right to euthanasia, and I'll sue you until you do it. And if you won't do it, get out!'

Her reply on exiting was 'Arthur, I can see how upset and angry you are, and I'm sorry that I can't give you what you ask for, but I can and would like to help you with your pain, and I'm happy to come back any time'.

He was visibly furious and she left the room. She felt that it was impossible to rationalise with someone who has lost their temper.

She clearly documented the conversation in his notes and fed back to the team and his wife. He was soon moved to clinical oncology in another hospital.

Key learning points:

- There will be times when you can't defuse someone's anger; they may be very attached to it and have their reasons and of course their own personalities. Arthur's request was unreasonable; perhaps he felt that he did have that right; maybe he was unaware of the law and maybe he was just too distraught to listen and reason that day.

- Sometimes, conversations are shorter than we would want them to be. I acknowledge the conversation was short, but her answer had to be clear – euthanasia is unlawful in the UK – and he had a right to end the conversation as he did. Continuing the discussion would only have caused him more distress and achieved nothing of any benefit.

People arrive in our care with a wide range of personalities and experiences for which we are not responsible. I'm sure that Lynn would have liked to have sat down with Arthur, listened to, and really understood his fears. She will have wanted to acknowledge and validate those feelings and reach a place where she could intervene to make life more bearable for him and his family by improving his pain management. That clearly wasn't possible. Sometimes, the only satisfaction you can get is knowing that you have done all you can, and that has to be enough.

I know that opinion does and will change in relation to assisted dying, and it is interesting to note that the BMA at its annual policymaking conference in 2022 delivered the results of the BMA survey of 2021. Members voted by a margin of 49% to 48%, with 3% remaining undecided, to approve a motion stating, 'This meeting believes that, in order to represent the diversity of opinion demonstrated in the survey of its membership, the British Medical Association should move to a position of neutrality on assisted dying, including physician assisted dying'.

This means that the BMA now has a neutral stance on assisted dying, mirroring the positions of the Royal College of Physicians, the Royal College of Nursing, and the Royal Society of Medicine.

Hospice UK, by comparison, published the following position statement on its website in 2018: 'Hospice UK has no collective view regarding the issue of whether the law should change to allow physician-assisted suicide. This is on the basis that the organisation represents over 220 member organisations, most of whom have not yet stated a clear position regarding this matter. It is different from a neutral position, which may imply an organisational perspective that has no interest in the outcome of the debate'.[4]

The whole ethos of hospice and palliative care, as defined by the World Health Organization, is that it 'intends neither to hasten nor postpone death'.[5]

This philosophy is a cornerstone of hospice care in the UK. If there were to be a change in the law relating to physician-assisted suicide in any of the four countries of the UK, Hospice UK believes that 'very careful consideration would need to be given to the effect it would have on patients and those important to them, to services, staff, and volunteers'.

I feel it is entirely reasonable to be scared of dying in distress, of the loss of independence and to feel strongly about the manner of our death. We do advocate choice, after all; we keep the patient voice at the centre of our plans for care in hard-working professional teams.

KATE'S STORY

Toby was 77 years old, bedbound, and very symptomatic from metastatic disease from a cancer of unknown primary origin. His wish was to die at home. His medical history included arthritis and poor mobility.

He had been sleeping more, been agitated regularly, hadn't eaten for 2 days, and was drinking very little. His family were of course worried about this.

Kate knew Toby's medical history well, including his intolerances and sensitivities to various medicines. She was aware of what had been tried already and what the drug contra-indications were in his case.

She knew that Toby was an undemanding and sweet-natured gentleman with the mental capacity to make decisions about his care. She knew from the discussions with his family and with other professionals that he was now in the final dying phase of his illness, and he was clearly struggling with lots of pain and agitation. His physical distress was obvious.

In his lucid moments, he was both intelligent and considered as he explained his wish for euthanasia. 'I don't want to suffer, and I don't want my family to suffer. This is not living, I'm stuck in a bed in agony with people I don't know washing me and cleaning me up (Wonderful as they mind.) This is no life, I'm done, I've lived my life and I'm ready to go. You must be able to give me something to see me off quicker. Please, Kate, you've been grand, I'll sign anything you want me to sign. My family agree, there'll be no drama, just send me on my way, please'.

Kate met his gaze and sat quietly for a moment. 'I hear you, Toby. I understand everything you say. Can you tell me what worries you most?'

Toby cried as he told her, 'Watching my family try to help when they can't – I'm in pain all over, nothing works, I get so panicky and then I can't breathe properly, then everyone panics, and I won't go in hospital. I'm not ending up tied to any bloody machines. I've seen that – nah, that's not for me, just send me off and have done.

'I can't even watch the game on the tele, my eyes aren't working so well, I was looking forward to the cup match, now I'm happy to miss it, I've had enough'.

Kate met his crying eyes and replied, 'Toby, I'm sorry but I can't see you off; it's illegal. No one can do that, and if you were to try that yourself, I'm sure you would end up in hospital on machines, and we don't want that.

'I've come today to change your medicines and how we give them. I'm doing that because you are right; things are changing, and I can see it's getting harder. Time is short Toby'.

'How short?' asked Toby immediately.

'I think we are looking at days now', Kate replied. 'I don't know exactly how many of course, but what I do know is that the change of medicines will help. We won't let the constant pain and those episodes of panic continue.

'If we switch you to injectable morphine for the pain, just like you've been on in tablet form, it will also help calm your breathing too, and if we add in my favourite drug midazolam, which will keep you and your muscles relaxed, I'm confident that we can make you sleepy enough to settle everything down. The cancer will make you unconscious soon anyway. You will be unconscious soon Toby, you won't be suffering. I'll start with the dose I think it is right for you, and we can top up with injections if we need to. And we'll increase the dose if we need to. We'll be using a syringe driver, Toby, a small machine with a battery that pumps the drugs in over 24 hours through a fine tube and tiny needle just under your skin. The community nurses will come to change it every day, and if you are struggling, they can come in to give you extra medicine.

'I know you're suffering now, but with these changes, you won't be. And it's important to be clear, Toby, that you won't die because of the drugs. I'm using them because you are dying and to support you to die peacefully.

'We have already completed the DNACPR form so there will not be attempts to resuscitate you; you are dying from a natural process. No hospitals and no machines.

'I'm going to write everything down on a form called an Advance Care Plan, and I'll leave it here and put it on the system so everyone knows what we have agreed today. No one wants you to be suffering, Toby; we want peace for you, and we will all work together to make sure that you die peacefully. Does that sound okay?'

Toby was quiet for a while, then said, 'Nothing has worked so far, so how do I know that this will?'

Kate replied, 'Because I'm studying everything we have done so far and working out the right dose for you. I'm not using baby doses, Toby; we know now that you need higher doses, and I'll use them because you need them, and if I have to increase them I will. I know these drugs, and I've heard you, Toby. I'm not seeing you off, but you will be sedated until you die'.

'Sedated?' asked Toby.

'Yes', confirmed Kate. 'Let me talk to your GP and your family, and I'll come back in. I've already asked the nurse to come in and give you an injection which will settle you until the syringe driver gets up and running. It will take about 6 hours to be fully in your system, so we will make sure we give you the drugs you need until then. After that, we can stop all the tablets you are taking, as they won't be helping now'.

Toby just nodded, and Kate went off to discuss the plan with the GP and family. When it had all been agreed and tasks were in place she returned to Toby to ask if he had any more concerns or questions.

He wanted her to go through it again, to assure him again that he would soon be unconscious, and she took the opportunity to advise him to have any important conversations now with his loved ones.

'As long as I'm out of it soon and my family is okay, I'm happy. I've done and said all I need to. I just want to go to sleep and not wake up'.

The community nurse had been and administered midazolam, and he was much more settled when Kate went back to him. She promised to call in the next day, and she made sure the family had all the right telephone numbers and information should they need them.

She updated his records on the shared clinical system and documented clearly in her own records. The Advance Care Plan was left in the home.

Toby died peacefully at home with his family 48 hours later.

There are some key points to highlight in that story, namely

- Kate had all the facts before her visit, and she had formed a clear clinical impression of his physical status. She was clear that the purpose of her visit was to adjust his medicine regime and adopt a new route of drug administration. The benefits of this are three-fold: It relieves some of the burden from the patient and family, it prevents them from having to repeat the events of the last few days, and it shows that as professionals we are well prepared, invested in their care, and working as a team. Also, knowing all the facts creates confidence in our own judgement, which is transferred to the anxious patients and the family. It also ensures that the discussion is focused on how the patient feels and what the right solutions are likely to be.

- She allowed him to speak, without interruption and showed she was listening. Body positioning and eye contact were crucial elements here.

- She acknowledged what he had said and told him that she had heard him, often repeating the phrases he had used.

- Kate was both calm and confident in her approach, which helps promote the same in the listener.
- His manner was clear and direct, and she replied in the same style, e.g., 'Sedated?' – 'Yes'. That was so important to him, a short answer was appropriate; no other words were necessary.
- Her explanation that she would not be euthanising him was given early in the conversation, and it was both clear and emphatic.
- Kate quickly moved on to the most important issue of why Toby felt this way and what he was scared of.
- She answered every question he asked and invited more.
- Importantly Kate was very clear that he wouldn't die from the use of these drugs but that she was using them because he was dying. This takes seconds to say kindly and prevents misconceptions being formed from the beginning. Also given that she had been asked to euthanise him, it is vital that she was clear that this was not her aim.
- The Advance Care Plan was left in the home because he had requested sedation, and it gave him reassurance. His family were also aware, involved and fully understood the rationale for Toby's and Kate's decisions.
- All communication with other professionals was prompt, clear, and recorded on the shared system and in her own records.
- Kate knew the value and pharmacology of the drugs that she advised. She could explain this and transfer her confidence to the patient and other professionals, and because of this, she was able to assure Toby that she would not be using sub-therapeutic doses.
- She revisited the existence and value of the DNACPR decision.
- Kate had heard Toby's wish to die and clearly had been concerned enough about his level of distress to intervene with a warning shot against his attempting suicide and outlined the likely consequences of doing this. The consequences part is so important. Most people won't have thought of this. They may expect an overdose to work quickly and effectively. Often it doesn't work, and with someone who was being so carefully monitored, it would have provoked a reaction and response that was the opposite of what Toby wanted, namely a hospital admission.

In summary, Kate was obviously an experienced specialist nurse who knew this patient and his pathology and physiology well. With experience comes confidence, clinical clarity and courage to take the right actions at the right time.

Of course, this is an individual case, and the treatment plan would not be appropriate for all or even most patients. We personalise care and base clinical decisions around that concept, which has to mean, as we know in palliative care, the whole-person approach including; physical, emotional, spiritual, and social elements.

In my view, one of the most important actions Kate took was to avoid the use of sub-therapeutic doses. As professionals, we all accept the required level of responsibility for using controlled drugs. Alongside that, we must take responsibility for using doses which are therapeutic doses both for the daily dose and for PRN doses. Appropriate training and education are vital to achieve the confidence to ensure this. This is particularly important when someone is actively dying when we have a limited chance to get the dosing right and could easily cause our patients and their family to lose confidence in our practice.

Prescriptions must be clear and allow for therapeutic doses, and PRN really should mean 'when necessary' and be used that way and at the appropriate dose with any ceiling dose for the drug clearly documented in order to support the clinician administering the drug.

Should the prescriber have any level of uncertainty, it is best practice to include communication with colleagues/peers in order to check out a recommendation.

If, as a profession, we are well educated, working safely in teams, communicating well and documenting accurately we should be able to apply confidence in our judgement therefore ensuring a symptom-managed death, as well as reducing the risk of a complaint or even litigation.

LOUISE'S STORY

Louise was a retired veterinary nurse with motor neurone disease. She was 58 years old and already coping with dysphagia, speech problems, and limited mobility in her right side. She had been happily married to Paul for 37 years and had 2 grown children with whom she had a close relationship. She was unable to care for her 3 grandchildren, who were all under school age.

She had valued her relationship with Danny, her palliative care nurse for 3 months, and as symptoms were progressing rapidly, she was sometimes very tearful during his visits but remained stoic despite her occasional distress.

At her recent visit, she told Danny she had a favour to ask him, 'Can you help me/ give me advice about assisted dying. I haven't made the decision lightly. We've discussed it as a family and my mind is made up, I just need your help'.

Using the same calm voice that Louise had used, Danny told her, 'That must have been so difficult to talk to your family about, and I see that you are sincere in your wish. I'm just so sad that that you feel so unhappy that you want to end your life. Is there something else I can do to help with your symptoms or care at home?'

'There may well be along the way', Louise answered. 'But we both know where this is heading; we know how I will die, and it will be awful. I don't want that for me or my family. I just don't, and I won't do it. So, there's no use trying to talk me out of it'.

Danny nodded and paused. Then he said, 'I can't advise you, Louise, although I appreciate and understand what you are saying, but as a professional, I can't be involved. The decision has to be yours, and any enquiries and research needs to be done by you or your family/friends. I know how well they support you. You are within your rights to do this, and I know that you will carefully consider all information about assisted dying before you commit yourself. It's important that you do that'.

After a moment's silence, Louise spoke. 'Okay, I understand. I'd just rather you told me what's what than the internet or a stranger'.

Danny replied, 'That's one big disadvantage of doing this, Louise; you will be dying with people you have only just met, even though your family can be with you. But it's a big decision that only you can make. When you have made the final decision, you need to ensure that your wishes are in writing and in terms of clinical advice; bear in mind that your mobility is deteriorating quickly; time is short, and you may feel too unwell to make the journey, sooner rather than later.

'I would also advise that we complete some documentation which will support you while you are here at home as well. Don't worry, you're not agreeing to anything that will prolong your life; the opposite actually. We know that cardiopulmonary resuscitation will not be a helpful treatment for you, and so I can help in completing your DNACPR form, and I would also advise that you complete an Advance Decision to Refuse Treatment, as this will give you back some control over what sort of care you want or don't want. This will protect you from interventions such as being kept alive on life support.

'You may even feel that when we have done that you feel reassured that your death will be comfortable without invasive intensive treatment. If not, then you can carry out your plans knowing that this legal document protects you until then. Can I leave the forms with you and I'll come back in 2 days to help you complete them? It's important that I talk to the team I work with, so they are in the loop when I'm not here, and your GP. Is it okay for me to do that?'

Louise nodded and smiled, saying, 'I'm still doing it though'.

Danny smiled back. 'And you can, Louise; that's your decision with your family. I will be looking after you until then, and you will have everything in place to ensure that your wishes are considered in every decision we make. It's just that legally I can't be involved in advising you or helping you with assisted dying. You've always been so organised – I'm so pleased you sorted out both your powers of attorney for health and welfare and finance; it does help your family and it's your views that matter now. So, I'll leave you with the information about the ADRT and I'll see you in 2 days'.

Key points from Danny's story:

- Clearly, Danny knew from the beginning of the conversation that Louise had considered this carefully, had discussed it with her loved ones, and had already decided that she would travel from the UK for assisted dying – which she had the right to do and the mental capacity to decide on. He acknowledges all of this and stated that he couldn't advise or support her with assisted dying early in the conversation.

- He was able to use her wish for control over how her life ended to talk about and advocate for an Advance Decision to Refuse Treatment. Clinically, there is no way of being absolutely sure how she will progress and at what speed or that other physical problems won't occur. The ADRT protects her on her journey, but it must be specific, witnessed, and recorded; he made that point well.

- Quite rightly, he encouraged her to keep her loved ones at the heart of discussions and decisions.

- He didn't try to dissuade her, whatever his views were. We don't know them, and neither did Louise.

- For some patients, the existence of an ADRT, an ACP, and a DNAR and a trusting relationship with the professionals involved in their care, is enough to ensure them that appropriate comfort measures will be taken at the end of life. For a small number of people, it isn't, and Danny supported both viewpoints well.

- He maintained his professional boundaries alongside clinical friendship.
- He assured her that there would be clear and timely communication with the wider team.

In my opinion, the way Danny handled this meant he could go home after work without worrying. Crossing the line professionally is guaranteed to keep you awake at night, whatever your good intentions.

As much as we may understand how Louise feels, and may think we would feel the same way, and possibly even wish that we could support and advise her (after all until this moment that's what we will have been doing). I assert that we can't be involved. In the UK, this is not part of our service; it isn't our role and could have serious consequences for us as professionals.

If you become known as the professional who advises patients on how to access assisted dying, you could and probably would, lose your job. You may find yourself in the media spotlight, unfairly tarnished for the support that you gave with good intentions. You have no way of knowing how the family will feel afterwards; they may blame you and accuse you of encouraging their relative to do this. It is possible that someone close to the patient vehemently opposes assisted dying. They may complain to your employer or registration body citing the advice that you gave as evidence of malpractice.

All swamps are messy, and my advice is to not be tempted to wade in this moral swamp. Your job description and your professional regulator protect you by being clear on what your purpose and boundaries are as a professional. And, of course, any assistance or advice you give to a patient which enables them to take their own life is unlawful and potentially punishable under UK law.

I know that many will agree not just with Louise's wishes, but with the proposal that assisted dying should be legalised in the UK, and in the future, it may well be, but at the time of writing, it isn't, and so our communication has to reflect that fact.

In Conclusion

It's always worth considering both sides of any argument thoroughly and to resist being influenced by individual cases. There is a plethora of research and information about assisted dying around the world. It is now part of the human story; it is legal in various countries, and the push for it to be legalised in the UK won't go away. The most important issue and the reason for this chapter is for you to be prepared to discuss this with those in your care with kindness, sensitivity, and, most importantly, clarity. Those attributes have to be in our toolkit; we will be needing them.

(See Chapter 8 for an advance decision to refuse treatment.)

> *TIP: Be compassionate and clear in your communication. Don't make decisions based on your personal views or accept responsibility for any advice/actions which may jeopardise your professional position.*

References

1. Resuscitation Council UK, Respect Process [internet], available at: https://www.resus.org.uk/respect
2. National Centre for Social Research, British Social Attitudes 34, Moral Issues. London, 2017; Available at: https://www.bsa.natcen.ac.uk/media/39147/bsa34_moral_issues_final.pdf
3. Hallows B, BMA moves to neutral stance on assisted dying [internet], British Medical Association, 2021; Available at: https://www.bma.org.uk/news-and-opinion/bma-moves-to-neutral-stance-on-assisted-dying#:~:text=Half%20(50%25)%20of%20surveyed,with%20a%20further%2011%25%20undecided
4. Assisted dying [internet], Hospice UK; Available at: https://hukstage-bucket.s3.eu-west-2.amazonaws.com/s3fs-public/2021-08/position-statement-on-hospice-care-and-assisted-dying-July2018.pdf [accessed March 2024]
5. World Health Organization, Palliative Care [internet]; Available at: https://www.who.int/europe/news-room/fact-sheets/item/palliative-care

14

It Can Happen to You and How It Feels When It Does

This chapter raises issues and challenges that will either have already happened to you or will happen to you at some point in your career. You, the reader, are also a potential (or actual) patient and, most probably, someone's loved one. When you are both a healthcare professional and a patient or loved one, in my experience, this can raise an extra layer of difficulty and anxiety. Such problems, if they arise, are not what we had anticipated, planned for, or even considered in advance. As professionals using healthcare services, we can often experience some benefits, but we may find it to be very stressful too.

It is important that I state clearly from the outset that we routinely navigate the same systems as everyone else in the same way, with generally little anxiety. Everyone in healthcare works extremely hard to provide excellent services, and as fellow professionals, we appreciate and value their investment every day.

However, at some point, there will be a personal crisis in our lives, be that sudden illness, a traumatic event, or the diagnosis of incurable illness. You may find yourself the patient, the main carer, or a spokesperson in these situations.

This chapter uses genuine case studies to demonstrate how it feels when we do experience the added stress of being a professional in situations where care could have been better. The case studies are real and illustrate the times when someone has been 'on the other side' of professional communication or had to 'fight the system' for their loved one.

Being the Patient

It is impossible to remove existing knowledge from your head, we are all a product of our experiences, and the chances are if your appointment is a routine primary care one, you will have already tried all conservative methods to solve the issue yourself. The first quandary, if it's the first time you've met this professional, is whether to declare your profession. It's easy to feel that stating it at the outset implies a sense of importance. It does not. I would argue that the professional you are consulting would rather you had an open conversation from the beginning, enabling them to tailor their communication style and clinical content accordingly. This negates the need for them to figure it out during the consultation by noticing the terms you use which demonstrate a clinician's level of knowledge.

DOI: 10.1201/9781003427377-14

LYDIA'S STORY

Lydia is an experienced General Practitioner (GP) and end of life care lead. She had endured neurological symptoms for 6 months, but no diagnosis had been made. She shares this story:

My consultant neurologist (whom I hadn't seen for 6 months or so) had last said it still seemed more like PLS (primary lateral sclerosis), the slow variant of motor neurone disease (MND) that doesn't involve the respiratory system. My husband and I went to the respiratory unit, I thought, to talk about my difficulty coughing – no, the consultation was about ventilation because 'I might need that soon'. BOMBSHELL and crap communication. I was totally unprepared and was just polite, and I said I didn't feel like talking about it as I had been assured that ventilation would not be needed. The embarrassed physiotherapist acknowledged that a diagnosis can change, and I came away with another bit of equipment called a 'cough assist' to use twice daily.

I am not stupid, and my medical friends have been nudging me towards the whole MND stuff, but I expected to hear it from my neurologist. So, a thousand tears later (from my husband as much as me) I am going for an overly optimistic lie-down. NO sympathy, please; it makes me cry and then affects my breathing.

We can learn from this and remember always to consider whether the patient is expecting a consultation which involves the breaking of bad news or the discussion of treatment plans. You will know that finding out what the patient has already been told and already understands is a key stage of breaking any bad news, and being told that you are facing the rest of your life dependent on assisted ventilation is definitely bad news.

In the physiotherapist's defence, they were right. Lydia did have MND, but she died before she actually needed ventilation. Their intentions were good, but the timing was awful, and the assumption that she was ready for that conversation or that it was needed at all was wrong.

Patients with a life-threatening illness often develop important relationships with their consultants and specialist teams, such as their specialist nurses. Understandably then, they expect the 'big' conversations to be had with those in that team. The physiotherapist, although extremely knowledgeable, was a transient relationship for Lydia. She was totally unprepared.

I want to be fair to them here, though; it is possible that the consultant neurologist found the prospect of breaking bad news to his medical colleague very difficult and that he had actually asked the physiotherapist to have this conversation. It's possible, but it was very unhelpful and potentially very damaging. Physiotherapists do such an important job, a crucial job for MND patients, but because this conversation was ill managed, Lydia didn't see them again.

I asked Lydia how this episode had left her feeling:
  I didn't want to seem 'arsey' as a professional. I was demanding, when my own loved ones were patients. I did mention that I found the way I had been told very difficult but it wasn't acknowledged and so I didn't feel I could push it.
  The term *health professionals* acts as a huge umbrella; a gastroenterologist does not know how to manage myeloma; a GP doesn't know how to do brain surgery. Just respect us but be kind.

Fellow professionals are likely to understand what it's like to do your job, or at least some aspects of it, they may also have had relevant clinical experience and education, know what good looks like, and be unforgiving if communication causes harm for them or their loved ones. Lydia's final piece of advice on this episode is clear, simple, and very important.

A patient or loved one may have disclosed that they are a healthcare professional, or you may have worked it out enough to ask them. However, you can't and shouldn't assume that they have the depth of knowledge that you do on the subject being discussed, and we know they may just have googled it, but they still don't have the knowledge to interpret the information accurately.

At the start of the consultation, specifically acknowledge a patient's profession and say, 'I am going to risk being seen as speaking down to you. I appreciate your job but I will speak in layman's terms. If you find that unnecessary, just tell me'. So, start with small building blocks and assess the rate at which they are taking them forward. Offer choices but also give your best advice, as it is so difficult to make decisions as an informed professional. It helps to respect their preferences when possible, of course, remembering that the responsibility for the final medical decision on whether to offer a course of treatment remains yours, and depending on the situation, it may be important to state this.

TONY'S STORY

Lydia also shared this anecdote with me:
  My mate (and fellow medic) Tony, who has had three bone marrow transplants for leukaemia is in hospital for investigation of abnormal liver function tests. We text several times daily and have a shared dark humour. He has by chance just sent a WhatsApp message saying:

> Ultrasound doctor was very entertaining. He said my liver looks delightful; which he explained means 'all OK in doctor speak'. I said, 'As long as you don't have a nice chianti waiting on the side, you can say my liver is delightful as much as you like'. He then left the room and came back in with a bottle of red wine! Very amusing x

Now that's good communication in terms of making the patient feel significant and engaged!

You will know that humour – often dark humour is a coping strategy and a binding force in healthcare. Members of the police, mortuary technicians, and funeral directors would all agree. I love the preceding anecdote and I know both doctors, who were both dying at the time this was written, both uber intelligent and helping each other cope. As stated, Lydia died recently, and I conducted the funeral service, and Tony, her doctor friend, spoke about a year of messaging each other and read a poem in tribute.

'Darkling Thrush' by Thomas Hardy

I leant upon a coppice gate
When Frost was spectre-gray,
And Winter's dregs made desolate
The weakening eye of day.
The tangled bine-stems scored the sky
Like strings of broken lyres,
And all mankind that haunted nigh
Had sought their household fires.

The land's sharp features seemed to be
The Century's corpse outleant,
His crypt the cloudy canopy,
The wind his death-lament.
The ancient pulse of germ and birth
Was shrunken hard and dry,
And every spirit upon earth
Seemed fervourless as I.

At once a voice arose among
The bleak twigs overhead
In a full-hearted evensong
Of joy illimited;
An aged thrush, frail, gaunt, and small,
In blast-beruffled plume,
Had chosen thus to fling his soul
Upon the growing gloom.

So little cause for carolings
Of such ecstatic sound
Was written on terrestrial things
Afar or nigh around,
That I could think there trembled through
His happy good-night air
Some blessed Hope, whereof he knew
And I was unaware.

MORE FROM LYDIA

The way bad news is communicated will colour the whole experience of palliative care for patients and their family. A rushed and blunt conversation will leave the patient traumatised and likely not trusting their doctor.

My dear friend Tony was told he had acute leukaemia in a consultation, which began, 'Brace yourself, we've got bad news'. 'We' didn't have it at all; my friend had it, and he changed consultant after he'd got over the shock, as he felt the relationship had got off to such a bad start that he didn't want or trust the way future news would be imparted.

I am a GP and learnt my diagnosis of MND on a telephone consultation when I was in the middle of surgery. I was so shocked I just thanked him and got on with my next patient's tale of woe. It wasn't until that evening, when telling my partner (now husband), that I broke down because I knew too well the burden he was going to have to bear and the inevitable grief. Being a medic is a double-edged sword. You know the end game but have difficulty translating into your life. Doctors carry on using 3-letter abbreviations for investigations and continue to suggest medications or treatments when actually what you need is more explanation to understand what the test involves and the pros and cons of medication. I have had experiences of both feeling unable to ask what a test will involve and not understanding what the results will actually say. But also, with medication, I have felt very at ease asking my palliative care doctors about the side effects and benefits of medication and making a joint, informed decision.

I have also realised that my training as a professional makes accepting being cared for very difficult. My stubbornness and determination can be seen as obstructive, and I feel I have failed when I need to ask for help and am treated as a lesser human being. I also feel the burden of grief that my friends and family are experiencing as they see me deteriorate, and that, more than anything, reduces me to hopeless tears (as writing this in fact just has).

Communication also relies on understanding the difficulties that people may have with the spoken word. My MND has taken away my ability to speak but not to hear or understand. I have an 'app' which speaks my pre-recorded voice, BUT this relies on patience. As my MND progresses my dexterity at typing worsens, so I am slow and make mistakes. If my husband is there, he can quicken things up considerably. The impatient doctor ploughs through and makes assumptions. I have to decide if it is a battle or skirmish and let the latter go. Pain is, at best, difficult to describe. I find it even more difficult to communicate my needs, so I often allow myself to be led down a path I didn't want to be on and agree to suggestions just to get out of the room. Likewise, people with hearing difficulties and poor cognition do struggle, so using appropriate language and available technology makes a huge difference.

Because of my interest in palliative care, I had picked up most of the MND patients in the practice as well as caring for some of them in the day centre of the local hospice. So I knew very well what was coming.

Before diagnosis, when my symptoms first started and my speech was starting to be affected, I was talking about it to the author of this book. 'As long as it's not MND, I'll cope with speech loss'. She very wisely acknowledged what I was saying but offered no false comfort, just support. So offer no false information but always offer hope.

It is difficult to find that hope in the darkest days and I find distraction is best. TV series (I am quite fussy), audiobook stories (I struggle to hold an actual book), Sudoku, and Wordle are daily addictions. I can no longer garden, play the piano or flute, sew, or paint, which were my greatest joys and distraction (especially when combined with a good audiobook).

It strikes me that the coping strategies that Lydia employs are based on maintaining connectivity and a sense of purpose. How we communicate, plan with, and guide people can support these elements, and her case study emphasises the value of doing so.

PAM'S STORY

I'm an end-of-life specialist palliative care nurse and had been struggling with head-aches. After trying the usual remedies, I visited my GP, and somehow (!) I failed the neurological exam. At the end of the consultation, the GP told me that she was sure I had a brain tumour, and she leant forward, held both my hands, and said, 'I wonder what you are thinking?'

Truthfully, my answer was, 'I'm thinking that you've just done a breaking bad news course and are practising on me'. I didn't understand how she could be sure without a scan. Clearly, she was worried. I saw the consultant neurologist the day after, who also said that 'I had a very good GP and that he was 99% sure I had a brain tumour'. He organised a scan for the following day (in case you are wondering, this was 20 years ago, when systems moved quicker). His parting words at the end of his consultation were 'If it's all clear I'll ring you myself; if I need to see you again, my secretary will ring you to make an appointment'. My reply was 'So, if it's your voice I'm OK, if it's your secretary's voice I'm in big trouble?' 'Ah' was his response.

I feel that being clinical does have its pros and cons, and I thought that the GP would have prompted me to cry and write my funeral plan, but neither consultation fazed me because I thought it was impossible to diagnose a brain tumour from clinical examination alone. At 58 years of age, I was more worried about them finding a neurological or vascular abnormality. My scan was clear (the consultant rang me himself), and to this day I don't know why I failed the neuro exam. To be brutally honest, I live in fear a bit of becoming symptomatic in later years and being told that it actually started 20 years ago but was too small for the MRI to detect. Oh the joys of being a healthcare professional!

Patients who are healthcare professionals aren't just likely to have some knowledge of pathology. They also know how the systems work in a way that laypeople don't, and it's helpful to bear that in mind too.

They might pick up the clues from the type of staff present at the consultation, a new specialist or a specialist nurse; how appointments are timed, e.g. urgently booked or booked at the end of clinic; the venue of the breaking-bad-news room (of course), and definitely the terms used, even the tone and body language used when discussing the planned appointment. As a reader, you will know that we can understand the meaning of such nuances in behaviour, but we might not always remember that a healthcare professional will too whenever they are our patient or our patient's loved ones.

Being the Loved One

JANE'S STORY

I'm an oncology specialist nurse with 20 years' experience. When my auntie Maureen died, I became the next of kin to my uncle Norman. They didn't have any children, they had led a very sheltered life, never made any demands on the system, paid their way, and always held anyone in the medical profession in high regard. They were part of a respectful undemanding generation, the 'pack up your troubles in your old kit bag' generation.

It was my brother who asked me to pop in and see what I thought. I hadn't seen my uncle for some time. I worked long hours, and my retired brother called in regularly to check on him.

I was shocked when I saw him. Clinically anaemic and frail, he'd lost weight, and the house smelled of faeces. He was polite to the professionals who knew him, and they had told him that he had lost weight because his wife had died. The diabetic nurse was happy because his blood sugars were stable. He wouldn't give me permission to contact anyone; he didn't want to cause trouble. Eventually I persuaded him and was there when the young GP visited; still he didn't want to go in hospital, and she concluded that she couldn't make him.

He was later admitted very unwell as an emergency to the surgical assessment unit. While I was with him, he was passing wind through his urethra, and I asked if someone would check to see if he'd fistulated. I was hoping for an ultrasound scan (he was the typical bowel cancer picture clinically). The nurse's response was that he had just broken wind, no need to worry.

It took 6 days with 6 different doctors and lots of pushing on my part to get scans and assessments before a surgical registrar told him that he had an unresectable rectal malignancy that he would die from. Unfortunately (and this had serious consequences), he didn't write anything in the notes. Norman languished on that ward, becoming frailer, and after 5 days of passing blood per rectum, he was given a transfusion. That was the only palliation he received, and every time I asked for a suitable treatment plan, I was told that I was the only person who thought that he was dying and that there was no evidence of a fistula despite the fact that I could literally hear it.

I know the staff thought I was hard work, but every day he deteriorated. He was moved to a discharge ward, and every day they told him that he was medically fit for discharge. He wasn't eating, was drinking only a little, and couldn't stand. He continued to lose weight and was doubly incontinent with blood in both his urine and faeces. He was clearly dying.

The plan was to discharge him to a care home, self-funded as a diagnosis wasn't written in the notes. In frustration and in front of the staff, I bleeped the registrar and asked him to come on the ward to write up his notes. He did, and then my uncle received funding for the care home.

He died 1 week later. From the beginning to the end, I had to fight the system for him. I didn't feel like I was dealing with professionals who cared until we met the funeral directors. It was an awful experience, where in my opinion no one cared enough to join up dots. I know that this is a sorry tale, but every word is true; maybe nurses get treated with less respect and more hostility than doctors, I don't know – but this all happened.

The GP who confirmed his death did not feel confident to confirm the cause of death, the notes sent from the hospital just weren't clear enough, and a postmortem was requested by the coroner, which showed rectal tumour and pneumonia. I'm glad that the case went to the coroner, whose bereavement nurse attached to the coroner rang me for feedback. She asked me to present the case to the hospital audit group, which I did, and they collectively assured me that they would not say you are medically fit to frail dying people, that they would keep that jargon to clinical teams where appropriate, but, alas it still happens.

The surgical registrar had also failed to refer to the ultrasound scan result which had revealed a fistula from a large rectal tumour. The CT scan report showed this also, and the coroner was the first person to read it.

Of course, there were lots of apologies for missing so many red flags.

At their request, I gave a lecture on how to diagnose dying, why it's important to join up the dots and to put their 'clinical deerstalker hat' on and how damaging it is to tell the family of a dying man that she is the only person who thinks he is dying.

It's a terrible story, I know, and hard to write when you are a nurse yourself and know how brilliant most professionals are, but as a reader, I'm sure that you will know that not every professional is brilliant at end-of-life care, and this reinforces the need for education – at every chance you get. It's likely that if you are reading this book then you already care very much about good communication in palliative care and you will do all you can to ensure that good communication skills are encouraged.

Of course, it's important to balance this torrid tale by saying that Uncle Norman did have some responsibility for his own health and communication decisions, and he made it very difficult; he had the capacity for decision-making and didn't give consent for Jane to act as his advocate. He just didn't want to be a nuisance, typical of that generation – that 'pack up your troubles in your old kit bag' generation.

The GP who initially visited could have said more to Uncle Norman in the way of professional recommendation. Yes, he had the capacity for decision-making, but as a layperson, he had no idea of the consequences of his decision; she could have pointed them out. We would expect this from a lawyer, car mechanic, or banker. I see professional recommendations as part of our job and especially important when someone risks making a detrimental decision due to lack of knowledge, knowledge that we have and can guide them with.

When the surgical registrar failed to write in the notes or speak to any staff caring for Norman, which caused huge problems down the line, Uncle Norman clearly didn't ask any questions himself and, at times, blocked communication too. However, no one asked him if he understood what anything meant, if he understood what would happen next.

Of course, not every patient wants to know bad news. It doesn't sound as though Uncle Norman did, but as professionals, we have to explain why we are making the decisions we are and not use meaningless phrases like 'medically fit'. As professionals, we know what that means, but it says something completely different to laypeople. He was totally unprepared and totally unsupported.

The burden was very much left to his niece Jane, and that may well have put strain on their relationship if he was solely relying on the information given by the professionals and feeling she was causing a fuss. To him, she wasn't a specialist nurse; she was his niece. To the staff, it seems as though they thought she was being awkward.

SEAN'S STORY

I'm an experienced community nurse and also the end-of-life care lead for the team I manage. I work alongside, and very closely with, the local palliative care team in my area of work, which is 25 miles from where I live.

I made the decision to move both my nonagenarian parents in with me; it was obvious that problems were starting to stack up both in mental and physical terms, and I wanted to avoid crises and decisions being made at crisis point. I knew very well the negative consequences of not planning well for the end of life. Following discussion with both my parents they had agreed that Do Not Attempt Resuscitation forms be completed and held with the GP and at home. A lasting power of attorney (LPoA) was done for both health and welfare and finance, and both my parents chose to complete an Advance Decision to Refuse Treatment (ADRT) in which both of them were very clear about their wish to die at home and avoid hospital intervention for the chronic conditions expected with old age. It was more detailed, of course, and these things develop over time, but that sets the context for my story.

Over a few months, at the age of 95 years, Dad started to decline physically and eventually ate less and less until he was eating nothing at all. He drank less and less and spent more time in bed. Eventually he couldn't get out of bed and slept a lot, and his lower legs became mottled. When awake, he was entirely lucid. I knew he was entering the dying phase.

As a family, we wanted to avoid an unnecessary postmortem, and because he hadn't been seen by a GP for over a month, it seemed prudent and indeed respectful to let the GP know that Dad was dying and to ask for a visit.

It was during the pandemic, and we waited for 7 hours for the GP to arrive. It was a locum who didn't know my parents, but I shared all the documentation with him.

He felt that Dad had a urinary tract infection because his temperature was 38 degrees and his urine output was low and very concentrated. On the basis of those two facts, he wanted to admit him for intravenous fluids and antibiotics. Conversely, I thought his temp was unremarkable for someone tucked up in a duvet, and his urine output was normal for someone who wasn't drinking anymore because they were, in fact, at the end of their life. Dad was very clear that he wouldn't go in hospital; he is old school and a very forthright northern bloke. My poor mum was heartbroken; after 70 years of marriage, she thought that the doctor was insisting that he would be taken in and would die alone in hospital (visiting was not allowed due to COVID-19 restrictions).

The GP and I had a discussion, and we disagreed as to whether my dad had mental capacity or not. Because my dad had replied, 'Bollocks', to his diagnosis and treatment plan, he felt that Dad didn't have capacity (I personally thought that it showed that he did). The doctor wanted to ask someone to come and check Dad's capacity **because** he had an ADRT – he had never seen one.

I explained all the paperwork clearly, saying that if Dad had the capacity to make decisions, then the ADRT was a legally binding document and was to be respected and his wishes upheld by law, but if the GP deemed that Dad did not have capacity, then the LPA was to be used as a decision-making framework; this would make me the decision-maker, and I was refusing his admission to hospital on his behalf.

He was baffled, and of course, he was acting as a locum for the practice, so he asked for another doctor to visit. We waited for another 4 hours. In the early hours of the morning, the second GP arrived, who, although he also wasn't familiar with Dad's case, fully understood all the paperwork, agreed with myself clinically, and all was well. He was both apologetic and frustrated.

Dad died peacefully at home 48 hours later. The medical certificate documented his cause of death as 'old age'.

The key learning point in this case study is that so many people, even professionals, don't fully understand the documents used in the end-of-life care legal frameworks in place. We must never assume that they understand.

You might think that because the documentation and laws with which you are familiar have been in practice for so long that everyone knows about them and understands them fully. As professionals, we can feel secure within our own clinical areas, use our own language, and forget to consider that other professionals, with vast knowledge in their own areas, are busy doing other things.

In theory, of course, we know this; palliative care teams are excellent and very proactive regarding education. However, this chapter is about 'how it feels when it happens to you'.

Sean was shocked that he had been forced to stand firm against the GP having done a 'belt and braces' job of planning and providing completed documentation. At the worst of times, Sean's stress and that of both his parents were increased.

I doubt that this GP as a locum felt that he had the authority to make such a big decision; he certainly didn't have the confidence, and he was acting very cautiously. It's reasonable, however, to have expected him to check with someone who did have the knowledge. He could have rung his local hospice, for example.

It's very true that any visiting healthcare professional may never have been educated about the decision-making framework relating to this case, or perhaps the education they have had, or the last time they used these documents was so long ago it is no longer at the front of their minds to draw on. GPs have so many responsibilities; by definition, their knowledge is general (although I appreciate that some do specialise in certain areas), so they cannot be specialist practitioners. I acknowledge the fabulous work some of them do to educate their teams and raise standards. In conclusion, out-of-hours end-of-life care presents challenges for clinicians; one phone call to the specialist palliative medicine consultant on call for the area by the locum GP could have made all the difference for this family.

Protecting Yourself

As a professional, your instinct is to care for people and be helpful when they ask you for advice. Often, it's okay to do this, straightforward even, such as the good old paracetamol and fluids for flu-like symptoms, or 'Don't ignore this; go to your GP', or 'Ring an ambulance now!'

However, there are other times when setting boundaries will protect you, and at those times, referring your family and friends back to their GP or specialist nurse is preferable. For one reason, they have the prescription pad, you don't, and even if you do, it is considered unethical to use it for family or personal friends not registered with your practice. Even giving advice could make you vulnerable; you could easily be blamed for adverse outcomes if you accept responsibility that isn't yours. The person asking you may not realise this. I am always clear that I do not have the medical notes and therefore could make a mistake.

Additionally, I know how hard it is to be the professional in the family, the one who they think knows everything and can fix everything, and let's be honest we want to. However, that comes with a cost, an extra layer of pressure at an already upsetting time. I appreciate that moving your mindset to a clinical template in your brain can be protective; it can even help you to cope with the chaos of the time. Conversely, it may not; it may feel 'too much', and you may need to say, for example 'In this situation I am just the daughter; I don't have all the answers, and actually I'm struggling too'.

Summary

I hope the case studies are useful and thought-provoking. It seems that this subject doesn't get mentioned in education, yet when you are faced with such situations, it can feel quite stressful and as demonstrated here can be the cause of bad memories for some people when they have been the patient or carer.

Instinctively, we try to be an undemanding patient/loved one, we fear being seen as difficult. This can lead to professionals not speaking out and not using their instinct and personal insight into the patient, and this can be a source of regret later.

It helps to be honest from the start about your profession and role because you can't change your experiences and knowledge base. Equally, be clear about your level of knowledge to ensure that the treating professional is not led to believe that you understand more than you do. Our level of knowledge varies enormously according to subject area and specialism.

Key Learning Points

Establish the communication style early on; be clear, sensitive, and respectful and agree together the level of involvement between the patient or loved one and the professional; and be clear on who is making the final decision.

Be honest about levels of knowledge and understanding. It's better to be 'talked down to' and have full understanding than be afraid to say that you don't understand. Only clear communication and agreed boundaries can stop this from happening. Having this conversation at the very outset prevents any dissatisfaction later or difficulty for the professional involved.

It is so important to be respectful and inclusive of patients or loved ones who are also healthcare professionals. It's possible that even though they are a professional, they ask to be spoken to and treated as a layperson due to the emotional strain of the situation. They may not want and may indeed be avoiding any form of responsibility.

It is prudent to always document the level of involvement the patient or loved one wants to have so that the next professional knows this and clearly document who wants to be the key contact. Always gain consent from the patient where needed.

> TIP: *As a patient or loved one – be honest and clear with the professional facing you; they want to get it right too.*
>
> *As a professional dealing with a patient or loved one who is also a professional, don't communicate in the style that would suit you; find out what style suits them.*

15

Frequently Asked Questions

The more faithfully you listen to the voice within you, the better you will hear what is sounding outside.

– Dag Hammarskjöld

The raised level of public expectation results in many questions being put to professionals. What seems simple science to a professional can be totally baffling to a patient and his family. The clinical reality can be hard for patients to hear, but a clear explanation is vital. The following list of questions contains both the common and some of the more difficult ones put to professionals, with tips and advice that may be useful to answer them. Suggested phrases are in italics.

- Why can't I just have a scan?

This is a common question; often, patients feel safer when they think that there will be regular scans, and they may request a scan more often than is clinically required. Patients usually think that everything shows on a scan. It may even be necessary to inform them that a tumour has to be big enough to be picked up on a scan and that clusters of cells are not detectable.

All treatments and investigations have a clinical basis. They are timed specifically for clinical reasons.

At this stage, it won't be useful. The doctor is an expert and will automatically order a scan according to the timing of your treatment.

There are other important ways of monitoring your illness, such as keeping a close eye on your symptoms and the blood tests we do also provide important information.

- Since they stopped the chemo, I haven't had a scan. How will we know what the cancer is doing?

We know that treatment will make things worse for you, not better. We don't do scans when treatment has stopped. It won't help you. What we will do is monitor your symptoms carefully and change your medicines when needed to keep your quality of life as good as it can be. You will probably feel so much better without the toxic treatments now and be able to enjoy life more. It isn't easy having regular hospital visits. We want to support you to have as normal a life as possible. Your community team will be monitoring you closely. It's important that we look after you at home, but there are still doctors and nurses available for you to see when you are worried.

- I don't understand. I had an appointment with the doctor 4 weeks ago, 2 weeks after my scan, and was told my last scan was stable. Why?

DOI: 10.1201/9781003427377-15

This is very hard for patients and their families to understand.

Sadly, your cancer has grown from when that scan was done 6 weeks ago. It wouldn't have been big enough to be seen at the time of the scan or have been big enough to cause you any symptoms.

- Then why not do scans more regularly?

Because it wouldn't help; if it wasn't big enough, we wouldn't have seen it. There wouldn't be enough time between scans to compare them and assess the effects of your treatment.

- You would think in this day and age that they would be able to do something; there must be some treatment?

I'm sorry to say that there are some diseases that have no cure, even today. Technology has improved, we do find problems earlier, and we can manage them for longer, but sometimes treatment can make it harder for you, not easier. And we won't give you treatment that we think will make it worse for you. I know that's hard to understand, but it is important that I am honest with you.

- Will it help if I pay for treatment?

This is a tricky one; there are some chemotherapy drugs that are available to patients with private health insurance but not those in the NHS. Avastin was an example. If a patient had private healthcare insurance prediagnosis of colon cancer, he may have received treatment earlier in his illness than he would have received it on the NHS, although this is happening less frequently. Within the UK, all medicines are assessed and recommended by the National Institute of Health and Clinical Excellence, in order to maximise benefit.

Usually, by the time patients ask this question, there is unlikely to be a treatment that will help them more than the treatments that are available in the NHS. Paying for toxic treatments, especially travelling to another country to acquire them, can be a disastrous plan.

No. The majority of experts work in the health service. Whilst some consultants may work from a private hospital, they have gathered their experience from working in the NHS. There is far more experience, knowledge, and support in the NHS. If you have a serious illness, you are in the best place, with the experts. All the treatments used have a lot of evidence behind them. Much of what you may read in the media about treatments refers to treatments that are in the very early phases of trials or aren't helpful for your disease. Your consultant has many years of experience. They specialise in medicine for your illness; the experts who will support you surround you. If I had your illness, I would choose to be cared for in the NHS.

- What do you mean, 'unknown primary'? You mean you don't know what kind of cancer I've got! Can you not find out?

The reality is that 30% of all cancers are classified as unknown primary. By the very nature of the disease, the cancer cell mutates to become unrecognisable, or very similar to lots of different types of cells. Sometimes a primary cancer remains undetectable on a scan, while its secondary deposits increase in size and distribution.

I know it's very hard to understand, but often we don't know where the cancer started. This is very common. We will do as many tests as we can to try and find out. Even if we never find out exactly where it started, we will try to offer treatment that will help you. We will try our best. If I don't know the answer, I will try to find someone who does. However, sometimes the most honest answer is, 'I don't know'. It is important that we are honest with you, and we will share all the information with you. You can ask questions at any time. We will always look for ways to make you feel better.

- A friend of mine's mum had cancer; she had radiotherapy. Why can't I have that?

Everyone has a cancer story, and patients often don't realise that cancer is hundreds of different diseases, rather than one. The histology (when available) and the stage of a cancer can provide clear prognostic indicators.

Every cancer behaves differently. There are more than 300 types. Any human or animal cell can become cancerous. Comparing breast cancer to lung cancer is like comparing bronchitis to diabetes, they are very different. It is common for friends to share their experiences with you, but comparing yourself to other people won't help you. Different cancers respond to different treatments. Your consultant is the expert in this type of cancer. He will prescribe the treatment that he thinks will help you most. Everyone responds differently to treatment. We don't know how well you will respond. It is very individual. Our job is to look after you and do the best for you. You will be closely monitored, and we will always be honest with you.

- Why can't you just cut it out?

It's a fair question and the first question asked to the clinicians. Many cancers are cured by surgery alone. The cancer may, however, be attached to vital organs or blood vessels or have already spread. The answer would depend on whether the question related to a primary or secondary cancer.

Primary Cancer

Your cancer is in a place where it can't be removed. It would be too dangerous to operate. Or – I'm sorry but it is impossible to get to the cancer without causing major damage to surrounding tissues and/or vital organs. It would be too dangerous for us to operate.

Or – I'm sorry but it would be too dangerous to operate, your body is not strong enough to cope with the anaesthetic or the surgery. It would be too great a risk for you. It wouldn't be safe or sensible to try.

Sometimes secondary cancers are entirely or partially removed. Consideration of whether this might be possible is an essential part of good palliative care to assess whether this is possible or helpful. An example would be the resection of an isolated secondary from a breast or colon cancer.

However, often when the patient has a burden of diffuse disease or a poor life expectancy, it may be neither possible nor helpful to operate.

Secondary Cancer

It wouldn't help to operate, as unfortunately, the cancer has spread to other places. Surgery would make things worse for you; it would take you too long to recover, and it wouldn't help at all. It isn't possible to remove all the cancer.

- Have I done something to cause this? Is it because I smoked?

Clearly the answer to this question depends on whether they have or not.

Non-Lifestyle Cancers

No. You have been very unlucky. It is nothing you have done, and you couldn't have done anything differently. It will help if you eat well, look after yourself, and give your body the best chance to fight the disease.

Lifestyle Cancer, Smoking-Related

Would it help you to know that? We know that smoking is bad for health, but it won't help to feel guilty. Guilt and pity are useless emotions. Try to avoid them if you can. We can deal with your illness now, and we will help you all we can.

If the patient insists on having a direct answer, then be clear. They may be parents who want to offer the best advice to their children.

We know that smoking significantly increases your chance of getting cancer. Yes, it is likely that smoking has caused your cancer. However, this doesn't make you a bad person or even a stupid one; it makes you an addict; there is a difference. When you started smoking, you didn't know what you know now. It is crucial that you are kind to yourself now. There are tough times ahead and beating yourself up won't help. We are always available to chat if it helps. There are millions of patients like you and lots of people to help.

- Why can't he have a liver transplant like George Best?

Your case is very different, and it wouldn't help you. Cancer is a totally different disease from liver damage due to alcohol. Cancer affects every system in your body and I'm sorry, but a liver transplant wouldn't work for you.

- Why have I been abandoned? Chemotherapy has been stopped, and now I have been cast aside and left to get on with it.

There is still a lot of support for you. Your consultant will see you again if needed. We can arrange that for you. Constant hospital appointments are tiring for you when you are not having treatment from the consultant; it isn't necessary to be waiting in busy clinics. Your community doctors and nurses will be looking after you now. You are in safe hands. I know it's hard when you get used to seeing certain doctors and nurses, but there is still a lot that we can do to help you. You haven't been abandoned. Often people feel so much better when they are not taking toxic treatments with all the side effects and clinic appointments. It does take some getting used to; it's a big change when your life has revolved around the hospital appointments, but you can enjoy a more normal life now and get more rest.

- If I'm not having any treatment, then the cancer will rampage, won't it?

Try not to imagine and torture yourself with graphic images, it's not like that. You may in fact feel so much better now the treatments have stopped, more like yourself again. Your body can rest and not have to cope with the side effects of the treatment. It wouldn't have been right to continue treatment that would have made you feel worse and wasn't helping you. We know that cancer cells can change, but we will watch things carefully and change your medicines regularly to keep your quality of life the best it can be. We are changing the way we support you, not giving up.

- They have always taken Dad in and sorted him out; why can't they do it this time?

I'm sorry, things have changed, and your dad is becoming overwhelmed by disease. The treatments we used before did help to manage the disease, but they will no longer help. He is too weakened by his illness now. It's very difficult to accept that the same treatment won't work again, but your dad's body isn't the same as it was. He is frailer, and his organs are not working as well as they were. I know that is hard to understand; we will do everything we can to help Dad feel as well as possible for as long as possible. We are not giving up, but we have to be honest about what we can achieve. It would be wrong to mislead you. Things are very different for Dad this time. You may have noticed things getting harder for him recently. Perhaps there are things he could do last week that he is struggling with this week? That is a sign that things are becoming much harder for him and his body is struggling to cope. We will provide medicines to help him with that.

- I am wondering whether to talk to someone else in the same position. Do you think it would help?

We can help with that; there are support groups that we can direct you to. It helps some people, but others don't find it helpful. You may meet people who seem to be coping better than you and that can make you feel that you are not coping as well as you should. Or you may be coping well and meet someone who isn't coping well, and that can set you back. Everyone is very different, even when they have the same cancer. They may be at a different stage, be having a different treatment, or be responding to it differently. But, as long as you remember that, it can sometimes help to talk to another patient who knows how it feels. Lots of patients have found it helps enormously but have sometimes felt sad when they have got to know someone who then becomes more ill. There are positives and negatives for you to think about carefully. You can go and try and see if it's for you.

- People go into hospices to die, don't they?

Sometimes, yes. Nowadays patients can go in for a short stay while their symptoms are sorted and then go home again. It is becoming less unusual for patients to go in and out regularly from a hospice. Yes, some people do die there, but they are very bright places, full of experts, and there is more chance of getting rest and much less chance of picking up an infection than in a hospital. It's a building full of experts who will try to get you feeling better and then get you home again as soon as possible.

- How long have I got?

How would it help you to know that? What would it change? It is difficult to know exactly; the honest answer is 'I don't know'. If you want an approximate answer based on my experience, I can give you one, but my advice is to sort your affairs; do the things you want to do and live your life as normally as possible.

Of course, if a patient demands specific timescales, it is fair and professional to give as much information as possible whilst repeating that it isn't an exact science. Whilst professionals don't have all the answers, they do know more than the patient. If a patient repeats the question, then he really wants the answer to the best of the professional's knowledge.

For example: *In my experience, patients with the same disease, in the same position as you, live at best 2 years and at worst 2 months. I really can't say where on that scale you will be. Rest when you feel tired and eat small regular meals. We will be keeping a close eye on you and helping you all we can to stay well for as long as possible.*

Writing a funeral plan is so helpful for families who struggle in the bereavement phase, dealing with administration and planning such an important event. It can help to add a sense of meaning to someone's life to be able to do this themselves.

- I want to plan my funeral, but it upsets my family if I talk about it so how to do it?

If you write your wishes down, it will really help your family when they come to plan your funeral. Making sure they know your wishes is a lovely, thoughtful thing to do. I can help you to write your funeral plan. First, you need to be clear whether you want burial or cremation, if you choose burial, do you know where you want to be buried? Is having a green environmentally considerate burial important to you?

What kind of service would you like, religious, just a few prayers, no religion, humanist?

Do you want a particular church or minster or non-religious celebrant?

Do you want a particular funeral director? Some people want limousines, and some people want a carriage and horses.

Is there particular route you want the funeral cortege to travel?

Have you thought about what kind of music you would like? It's usual to have 2 or 3 songs or hymns.

Have you any favourite poems that you would like to be read?

Is there anyone that you would prefer to read the eulogy? (A tribute to you)

Do you want a wake, and have you thought about where you would like it to be held?

Are there any documents or notes that you have left for your family/friends to help them plan the funeral, where are they?

Are there any people that you would direct your funeral planner to, someone who knew you when you were young, for example?

- You must be used to this. Am I normal?

Yes. The range of normal is wide. Everyone is different, so I don't get used to it; this is the first time I have met you. My job is to support you as you are. Comparing yourself to anyone else won't help you.

- Do you think I have time to go on holiday?

This question may be from the patient or the relative and may come at a variety of stages of the illness.

From a Relative in the Patient's Dying Phase

Time is now short for your mum, things are changing, and how quickly they will change is not always predictable, but we will do our best to keep you informed. If it is very important to you to be here when Mum dies, then I would advise you to stay. I can't predict just how long Mum will live, but if you would feel guilty afterwards if you weren't here, the best decision is to cancel your holiday. Our doctor can complete the forms needed for your medical insurance.

If you are content with the knowledge that your mum might die when you are away, then I suggest you chat to Mum and the rest of the family (if applicable) and go on your holiday knowing that

Mum is well cared for. I will give you some contact numbers in case you want to keep in touch. If you want us to contact you during your holiday we can, or we can talk on your return.

From a patient. Of course, the answer to this question would depend on the stage of illness and where the patient was planning to travel to. Travelling to the United States, Africa, Australia, or the Middle East from the UK can be hazardous, given that there is often no reciprocal agreement to provide or fund healthcare. Conversely, trips within the UK or Europe are less problematic for citizens of the UK.

If you are staying in this country, or going to Europe, and your consultant is happy with the timing of your holiday, by all means. If we need to talk to professionals where you are staying, we can do that, and we can also give you a letter to get your medicines through customs. Do you feel well enough to travel? It may not be the same as your last visit; do you think you would still enjoy it as much?

- Am I dying? (from a dying patient)

Things have got much harder, haven't they? Yes, I am sad to say that time is now short. (PAUSE; allow the words to sink in.) Patients need time to gather their thoughts and feelings and to name their emotions. They ask because they want to know the answer. If they didn't want to know, they either wouldn't ask or would provide the answer they wanted as part of the question, for example – 'Am I dying? No, I know I'll be okay; it's just a bad day'.

How bad do you feel; do you want to talk about that?

- Are you not giving me any treatment because of my age?

Whilst there are times when a patient's age and in particular his co-morbidities are clinical factors, often, especially in oncology, a patient's suitability is assessed from his performance status. His level of activity and mobility provides more useful information than age. The following statements may apply.

As you get older, your kidneys, for example, don't work as effectively, your body wouldn't be able to cope with this treatment, and if we gave it to you, it would make you really ill, and it wouldn't help.

No. It isn't because of your age. This treatment wouldn't work for your disease (at this stage of your disease).

- She doesn't eat any more. Is she starving to death?

This is a common question when a relative is faced with a loved one who can no longer eat normally. They imagine that the patient is starving to death and that he would live longer if only he ate more. It causes one of the most common tensions in the family home. Patients may feel inadequate, embarrassed, frustrated, guilty, and ashamed. Constant discussions about meals are wearying and burdensome. Family members may feel helpless, since providing food is seen as such a crucial role when someone is ill. They want the patient to continue to enjoy the psychosocial benefits of meals. Both the patient and his family may try harder and harder and become trapped in a vicious circle. Some of the following dialogue may be useful to help relieve that tension. Be aware that there is no ethical or legal difference between not starting or stopping a treatment which you know to be unhelpful and then stopping one which no longer helps the patient. Within the context of palliative care, this is true also of the role of artificial nutrition or hydration. The different statements can be applied at different stages of the patient's illness.

It is normal to lose your appetite/lose weight. It is part of the disease sadly. Most patients are unable to eat enough to avoid weight loss.

I would advise you to stop weighing yourself. It won't help. Eat what, when, where and as little or as much as you want. Because your body is behaving in a different way, weighing yourself may cause you constant upset.

I know you feel that this is the one thing that you can do to help, but constantly suggesting or asking about food can make him feel worse.

Allow him to feel hungry and then he'll tell you what he feels like eating.

Small, regular meals are best. A normal-sized meal will be too much most of the time.

Obey the messages your body gives you; if you feel something may make you sick, it probably will.

The illness prevents the body from absorbing the nutrients and alters the way food is metabolised. The illness causes protein and muscle to become wasted – that's why you're weaker.

It is impossible for him to eat enough to make him as well as he was.

Appetite stimulants and food supplements may affect a patient's appetite, weight, and quality of life, but they do not prolong life in the terminally ill.

When someone is bedbound from this illness they don't feel hunger often. When they do, they need only small amounts of food and fluids to satisfy them.

- Surely, he needs a drip (IV fluids) up or something?

Many of the above statements and explanations can also be transferred to this question. It may be valuable to add the following.

At this time the body does not need the same amount of fluid and would be unable to cope with too much. It would cause too much of a burden on the system and make him feel worse; it could make breathing harder for him. He doesn't feel thirsty in the same way as before. It is okay to offer sips of fluid when he asks and if he can swallow safely. The most important thing is to keep his mouth clean and his lips moist. This helps a great deal to increase comfort.

- When the morphine starts, he will die quicker, won't he? It's the beginning of the end?

Often patients and their families have had some experience of morphine. They may have misconceptions relating to addiction and that its use can hasten death. Morphine is a good drug. It remains the first-line treatment for pain in palliative care.

It is commonly used and should be well understood by those who prescribe or suggest its use. Many patients have already used various codeine preparations prior to the prescription of morphine. Transferring them to morphine is therefore a sensible and effective step in achieving pain control. When patients are informed that they are not opioid naïve and that their bodies are already used to a dose of morphine, they relax about its use significantly.

Addiction does not occur when morphine is used for pain control; the problem does not apply to palliative care patients. It's important to be clear about that and that syringe drivers are used in the dying phase because the patient is dying. This may have to be stated explicitly.

We are using a syringe driver because Dad is dying and can't swallow his medicines anymore. He will not die quicker because of the syringe driver; he will simply die more peacefully. It can seem that someone dies because a syringe driver is started; in fact, they were dying before it was used. It's the best way to support him and to keep him comfortable. Is there something you would like to ask me?

- How will I know he is dying?

You will see the changes. He will stay in bed more and eat and drink less. Often people slip into unconsciousness at the end in a peaceful way. You will notice the changes in the breathing during the final phase. Don't worry, the doctors and nurses around you will see the changes and advise you all the way through.

- What will happen? Will I be in pain or just go to sleep?

Usually dying is a peaceful process, whereby the body slows down and gradually stops. It is likely that you will be unconscious at the end, and we will use medicines that we know will keep you comfortable. We won't allow you to be in pain or have breathing problems.

- What will be the thing that actually kills me?

Death is caused by an accumulation of damage. Gradually the cancer will stop your vital organs from working effectively. As your body becomes slowly overwhelmed, your organs will function less well, slow down, and stop. This will be a gradual process and we will support you with medicines that will help during this time.

- Why can't you just give him something? You wouldn't let a dog suffer like that.

It never helps to compare a human to a dog, but it doesn't help to say that. It is a thought that many people have, because of the pain they are in whilst watching the change and suffering of those they love.

I know this is very hard for you. It must be the worst of times, and I understand that you don't want him to suffer. We will do all we can to keep him comfortable and prevent suffering. It is against the law to give anything that will shorten life. However, I promise that we will not do anything to prolong suffering. We will help him to die naturally and as peacefully as possible.

- Who do we tell when he dies? What do we do?

If a patient has died in hospital, the next of kin will have to collect the death certificate and make an appointment to register the death. The undertakers chosen by the family can collect the body from the hospital mortuary. If a postmortem has been requested, the death certificate and the body can only be collected after this has taken place.

When patients die in their own home, it is their GP who will provide the death certificate. If the death has taken place at night or over the weekend, the out-of-hours doctor is required to visit to verify the death, and the body can then be removed by the undertakers. On the next working day, the patient's GP is required to issue the death certificate. Out-of-hours doctors can only confirm death; they cannot certify a cause of death in the UK. If the patient has not been seen by his GP during the last 14 days of his life, by law in the UK (28 days in Northern Ireland), a postmortem is required. This will hopefully have been avoided by the provision of good end-of-life care and professional planning. There are helpful leaflets which will guide the bereaved through the bureaucratic process of death registration and useful websites that professionals can direct them to.

It is valuable to reassure the family of how helpful and professional the undertakers are. The public tends to see the undertaker arrive at the funeral with the coffin and have no idea how much important work they do. Reassuring them of how supported they will feel by this profession can relieve stress from the situation.

If a postmortem is required, this will usually have been already discussed with the patient's family.

If a patient died suddenly or had not been seen by a doctor in his last illness, the law requires a postmortem. In those circumstances, the body belongs to the coroner. The coroner and their assistants are highly skilled at communication with the bereaved; they will keep the family informed in a kind and businesslike manner. If the family are in this position, it is a kindness to reassure them of how professional and helpful the coroner's office can be. For many people, these are new experiences, and they are therefore learning facts at a time when they are under huge emotional strain.

If the deceased is to be cremated, then two doctors, one of whom cared for the patient during his illness, must sign the death certificate. A doctor who did not know the patient, and has no clinical association with the first doctor, must complete the second part.

- Yes, but you don't know how this feels. This has never happened to you, has it?

Patients and their families have no idea what has and hasn't happened to a professional. Each individual is a product of their own experiences. A professional does not have to give any personal information unless it feels comfortable to do so.

I have known illness and death personally, but I am here to understand your situation and help as much as I can. I have cared for many people in these circumstances, and I will use that experience to help you whenever possible. Is there something that you feel I could help with today?

> TIP: *Asking whether there is 'something' a patient or his family may want to ask is more likely to elicit a positive response than asking whether there is 'anything' they would like to ask.*

16

Looking after You

Life does not cease to be funny when people die any more than it ceases to be serious when people laugh.

– George Bernard Shaw, Irish dramatist and socialist (1856–1950)

Working with palliative care patients is both rewarding and emotionally costly. It is impossible to engage enough and provide the necessary emotional investment without there being a cost to the experience. The challenge for professionals is how to manage that cost.

Realistic Objectives

It helps enormously for professionals to set realistic objectives. Professional 'burnout' is far more likely to occur when professionals set themselves objectives that cannot be achieved. Palliative care patients, by definition, have a life-threatening disease, and the vast majority of them will die. All patients will have endured various minor or self-limiting illnesses during their lives, but they will only die once. That a professional can have a positive impact on their death is truly rewarding.

Cure to Comfort

Dying patients die. Managing how they die and improving the experience for the patient and his family is a worthwhile and entirely achievable goal. The emphasis of care therefore shifts from cure to comfort. Providing that comfort includes a more technical approach than it did years ago. Many treatments are used palliatively; radiotherapy, chemotherapy, surgery, and anaesthetics are often used. The comfort agenda dovetails effectively with other specialties.

The Science and the Art

The clinical sciences coexist with the art of caregiving. Patients require and deserve both sets of skills and knowledge. Concentrating on the clinical aspects can be both beneficial to the patient and protective for the professional. If a patient is to be offered sage, accurate

DOI: 10.1201/9781003427377-16

advice, the professional has to engage in and understand the clinical facts. This part of clinical practice demands total concentration, so much so that at times, the professional is required to step away from the obvious emotional impact on the patient. Indeed, understanding the clinical situation and prognosis may provide important indicators of how the patient is likely to be feeling in the future. This allows the professional time to plan the support that will be needed, and crucially, to absorb the emotional impact of bad news herself. Whether it is a patient already known or a name on paper, it is a person with relationships who matters.

Strong and Soft

Professionals are usually sensitive people, 'soft' some may say. Soft, however, does not translate to weakness. They are also usually 'strong' too: soft enough to anticipate the needs of others and strong enough to cope with and meet those needs.

All professionals in healthcare have phases when they have been hurt and made mistakes and have usually had times when their emotions got the better of them. Those troubling times provoke an important adjustment phase and, crucially, a painful method of learning about both the job and themselves.

Adjusting to the Work

This phase of adjustment and the lessons learnt benefit every patient that the professional meets thereafter. Professionals who block that painful adjustment stay in the first phase, and because it is a painful place to be, they employ 'blocking tactics', such as ignoring the cues from the patient, changing the subject, and redirecting the dialogue. Caring comes with a cost; if the cost feels too great, it is human to engage to protect oneself. But this tactic impedes both personal and professional growth.

Professionals working in health care tend to be very self-aware. It is impossible to hide from oneself or close team members. In an emotionally charged environment, people's personalities and their weaknesses and strengths are revealed on a daily basis. That professionals see sadness and courage as part of their everyday life affects them massively. The level of self-awareness is both positive and accumulative. The job gets easier with time. It never gets less sad, but it does get easier when a professional knows her strengths and weaknesses and has engaged closely with a trusted team to work in a synergistic way.

Only amateurs consider themselves indispensable. Palliative care is a team activity. There is always someone else to help the patient. The need for constant availability doesn't exist for every professional within palliative care; a palliative care professional is not the key worker.

Communication dilemmas do not have the urgency that is often attached to them in other clinical settings. There is usually time to think, consider, and discuss with others before responding. Professionals can therefore reduce the stress on themselves by remembering this and allowing themselves some thinking time. In addition, there is often someone with greater knowledge or skills to help. Knowing when to say, 'I don't know', and asking for help is a great form of self-protection and learning.

Professionals as Human Beings

Every professional has her own family and worries. Life still hurts in other ways, and seemingly small things can cause irritation and anxiety; this is normal. Professionals still have every right to feel their own feelings; it's inevitable. Caring for the dying does not sanctify anyone, although it may alter perspective! For example, a teenager with a dramatic response to a headache may get little sympathy from a parent who has spent the day with palliative care patients. This is understandable and, whatever a dramatic teenager may think, entirely forgivable. It is so important that professionals are kind to themselves. Working and home life are often difficult at the same time; it can feel as though one's whole life is about giving and meeting the needs of others.

Having hobbies and as much pleasure as possible is vital; the 'empty tank' of an exhausted professional needs to be filled. It really doesn't matter what those hobbies and pleasures are. Whether it is watching soap operas and drinking red wine, walking, swearing, laughing, or doing absolutely nothing, a busy professional should do it, just do it, because each person knows what they need, they have no doubt learnt the hard way to leave work behind and be themselves.

It takes time to 'swap heads' – for example, to leave the physiotherapist behind and become a mum. The journey home can help. Music can help and sometimes it's silence that is needed. Every day may require a different strategy. There may be times when endless superficial 'chitchat' is just what is needed and other days when it would be too irritating to endure. If a professional obeys her own thoughts and instincts, she is likely to make the right choice, and choices will vary according to mood.

It is imperative that professionals are both kind to and forgiving of themselves. Guilt is a useless emotion. If a professional snaps at her children when she gets home, it's normal, it's okay, and it's life – her life! Professionals do not own the patient's or his family's feelings, they have lives full of their own, and they will have their own experiences of loss and heartbreak.

The Value of Humour

Laughter is sustaining and binding. Even laughter at the macabre can and does relieve stress. It's allowed! In private, with similar-minded professionals, it is one of the best ways of dealing with the emotional onslaught within palliative care. It helps to embrace it, create it, and feed off it. It is both human and protective.

> *TIP: As a professional be highly self-aware, take every opportunity to be yourself, do whatever helps, and laugh every chance you get.*

17

Conclusion

After medicine has finished doing all that it can, it's the stories that we want and, finally all that we have.[1]

As the author, I have chosen to add a personal touch to the conclusion. It is my attempt to talk to the reader directly. More than anything, I hope that it is my love of palliative care that has come across to the reader. At this point, I am no doubt preaching to the converted. The professionals reading this book will inevitably be those who want to learn more about this subject and already care enough to work hard to hone their skills. Such is the way of education in healthcare.

I write from my experience; the fact that I have lots of it, I feel, makes my writing credible. That I have chosen to avoid theories/models and a long reference list I think makes this book readable. My aim has been to acknowledge the extraordinary whilst remembering just how ordinary I am. I have been an ordinary specialist nurse and mum, an ordinary hospice chief executive and daughter, and I am an ordinary funeral celebrant, and Grandma who knows how to listen to tell a story about those who matter to us all, our patients and their families.

It is my belief that staying true to ourselves and cherishing our own spirit is crucial to enjoying and flourishing within palliative and bereavement care. There will always be new technologies and drugs, new systems and pathologies to learn. Yet, ultimately, our patients will all die in the same way; however different the route to their death may be, they will die when their heart stops beating and sending oxygen to the brain. We choose to be there alongside them.

Kindness and common sense are attributes as valuable as academic achievements. I would encourage the reader to consider that, within an environment of ever-increasing demands and stresses, describing and validating what you do is more important than ever, to consider and expand on what it really means to be caring and just how much difference it makes.

Healthcare workers are often strong self-aware individuals, not easily daunted by the challenges of modern life. Dramas and soap operas could never represent what we see and help with on a daily basis.

As sensitive detectives, we weave our way through information, knowing when to intervene, and how to lead probably the most important discussions of a person's life. It is a huge responsibility. Only our enthusiasm and tireless commitment to making a difference sustain us and provide the confidence needed to continue.

Allowing the patient to verbalise his feelings, in his own way and time, is absolutely crucial. So often professionals assess the problem and dive in too quickly with advice, missing out on the most informative part of the conversation. The patient's and his

DOI: 10.1201/9781003427377-17

family's feelings offer so much information about what they understand and hope for. This is vital information, which will enable the professional to meet the needs of a wide variety of people.

The body may be healed by medicine, but the mind may be healed by a story. Thank you for reading some of mine.

Reference

1. Saunders L. *Diagnosis – dispatches from the frontline of medical mysteries.* London: Icon Books; 2009. p. 251.

Index

Pages in *italics* refer to figures and pages in **bold** refer to box (case study or tip).

Printed in the United States
by Baker & Taylor Publisher Services